Publish and Flourish
A Practical Guide for Effective Scientific Writing

Publish and Flourish
A Practical Guide for Effective Scientific Writing

Editor

Amar A Sholapurkar BDS MDS FAGE
Reader
Department of Oral Medicine and Radiology
Manipal College of Dental Sciences
Manipal, Karnataka, India

Forewords
Prof K Ramnarayan
Prof Shobha Tandon

JAYPEE BROTHERS MEDICAL PUBLISHERS (P) LTD
New Delhi • Panama City • London

Published by
Jaypee Brothers Medical Publishers (P) Ltd

Corporate Office
4838/24 Ansari Road, Daryaganj, **New Delhi** - 110002, India
Phone: +91-11-43574357, Fax: +91-11-43574314
Website: www.jaypeebrothers.com

Offices in India

- **Ahmedabad**, e-mail: ahmedabad@jaypeebrothers.com
- **Bengaluru**, e-mail: bangalore@jaypeebrothers.com
- **Chennai**, e-mail: chennai@jaypeebrothers.com
- **Delhi**, e-mail: jaypee@jaypeebrothers.com
- **Hyderabad**, e-mail: hyderabad@jaypeebrothers.com
- **Kochi**, e-mail: kochi@jaypeebrothers.com
- **Kolkata**, e-mail: kolkata@jaypeebrothers.com
- **Lucknow**, e-mail: lucknow@jaypeebrothers.com
- **Mumbai**, e-mail: mumbai@jaypeebrothers.com
- **Nagpur**, e-mail: nagpur@jaypeebrothers.com

Overseas Offices

- **Central America Office, Panama City, Panama,** Ph: 001-507-317-0160
  e-mail: cservice@jphmedical.com, Website: www.jphmedical.com
- **Europe Office, UK,** Ph: +44 (0) 2031708910
  e-mail: info@jpmedpub.com

Publish and Flourish: A Practical Guide for Effective Scientific Writing

This book has been published in good faith that the material provided by the contributors is original. Every effort is made to ensure accuracy of material, but the publisher, printer and editor will not be held responsible for any inadvertent error (s). In case of any dispute, all legal matters are to be settled under Delhi jurisdiction only.

First Edition: **2011**

ISBN 978-93-5025-346-5

Typeset at JPBMP typesetting unit

Printed at Rajkamal Electric Press, Plot No. 2, Phase-IV, Kundli, Haryana.

Dedicated to
My Parents
and wife

CONTRIBUTORS

Wilfred C G Peh
MBBS (Singapore), MHSM (Sydney), MD (Hong Kong), DMRD (London), FRCP (Glasgow), FRCP (Edinburgh), FRCR (UK)
Advisor and Immediate Past Editor,
Singapore Medical Journal
Clinical Professor, National University of Singapore
Senior Consultant and Head
Department of Diagnostic Radiology
Khoo Teck Puat Hospital, Singapore

Kwan-Hoong Ng
BSc (Aberdeen), PhD (Malaya), MIPEM (UK), FInstP (UK), DABMP (USA)
Editor, Biomedical Imaging and Interventional
Journal
Senior Professor, Department of Biomedical Imaging
University of Malaya
Malaysia

Fatema Jawad
MBBS (Dow Medical College, Karachi) MCPS (College and Physicians and Surgeons, Pakistan) FRCP (Edinburgh)
Editor-in-Chief
Journal of Pakistan Medical Association
PMA House, Aga Khan 111 Road
Karachi, Pakistan

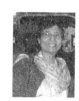

Prakash Mungli MBBS MD
Associate Professor in Biochemistry and Genetics
St Matthew's University, School of Medicine
Grand Cayman, Cayman Islands, BWI

Nirmala Rao BDS MDS
Dean
Professor
Department of Oral and Maxillofacial Pathology
Manipal College of Dental Sciences
Manipal, Karnataka, India

Keerthilatha M Pai BDS MDS
Associate Dean
Professor and Head
Department of Oral Medicine and Radiology
Manipal College of Dental Sciences
Manipal, Karnataka, India

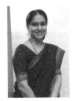

KL Bairy MBBS MD PhD
Professor and Head
Department of Pharmacology
KMC Manipal
Director, Manipal Center for Clinical Research
Manipal, Karnataka, India

Shailesh Lele BDS MDS
Principal, Professor and Head
Department of Oral Medicine and Radiology
Sinhagad Dental College and Hospital
Pune, Maharashtra, India

Ranganathan Kannan BDS MDS MS (Ohio) PhD
Department of Oral and Maxillofacial Pathology
Ragas Dental College and Hospital
Chennai, Tamil Nadu, India

Shreemathi S Mayya MSc MEd PhD
Associate Professor
University Department of Statistics
Manipal University,
Manipal, Karnataka, India

Kandaswamy Deivanayagam BDS MDS
Professor and Head
Department of Conservative Dentistry and Endodontics
Meenakshi Dental College
Chennai, Tamil Nadu, India

Vijay Prakash Mathur BDS MDS
Assistant Professor
Department of Pedodontics and Preventive Dentistry
Center for Dental Education and Research
All India Institute of Medical Sciences
Ansari Nagar
New Delhi, India

Sumanth Prasad BDS MDS
Professor and Head
Department of Public Health Dentistry
ITS, Dental Center for Dental Sciences and
Research Muradnagar
Delhi, Meerut Road
Ghaziabad, Uttar Pradesh, India

Vidya KM BDS MDS
Senior lecturer
Department of Oral and Maxillofacial Pathology
Ragas Dental College and Hospital
Chennai, Tamil Nadu, India

Ashutosh Sharma BDS MDS
Consultant, Pediatric and Special Care Dentistry
Shams Moopen Dental Practice (DM Healthcare)
Dubai Marina
Dubai (UAE)

Amar A Sholapurkar BDS MDS FAGE
Reader
Department of Oral Medicine and Radiology,
Manipal College of Dental Sciences
Manipal, Karnataka, India

FOREWORD

I am delighted that Dr Amar Sholapurkar has embarked on this venture of bringing out such a much-needed book on *'Publish and Flourish: A Practical Guide for Effective Scientific Writing.'* Any scientific work must be published and therein lie the pitfalls. I must congratulate him for the timeliness and the content. At this time when, scientific writing is becoming even more daunting with 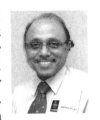 the plethora of scientific journals, it is fitting that this book addresses some very foundational issues pertaining to scientific writing. The comprehensive coverage of topics in the book will provide all the necessary information for the fledgling scientific writers as well as to the more experienced ones. It is not always easy to get all the information pertaining to scientific writing in one place; this book is indeed a laudable effort in that direction. The contributors, with their extensive experience in scientific writing, have lucidly articulated their viewpoints on very many subtle issues associated with writing science. This book is a must-read for anybody who takes scientific writing seriously, systematically and scientifically. Let this book make scientific writing more enjoyable and worthwhile.

Prof K Ramnarayan
Vice-Chancellor
Manipal University
Manipal, Karnataka, India

FOREWORD

I am extremely glad to pen down a few words about this conscientiously written book titled *'Publish and Flourish: A Practical Guide for Effective Scientific Writing'* which is a unique and pioneering attempt by a very young and dynamic faculty, Dr Amar Sholapurkar.

A critical aspect of the scientific process is the reporting of new results in scientific journals in order to disseminate that information to the larger community of scientists. Communication of one's results contributes to the pool of knowledge within our discipline (and others) and very often provide information that helps others interpret their own experimental results. An objective of organizing a scientific research paper is to allow people to read one's work selectively for which excellent writing skills are essential for effective communication.

This book is indeed comprehensive with well-compiled chapters which are formatted in an easy sequence. The author has made a sincere and systemic approach to present succinct panorama of various aspects on how to write scientific paper to fulfill the long-term need of a concise book in this field. I am sure that owing to its simple language and in-depth explanation of every section, this book undeniably be used by all those students and faculty members who are craving to mark a niche in academics.

On behalf of all the students and fraternity of MCODS, Manipal, I take this opportunity to congratulate Amar A Sholapurkar for this commendable work and hope that we would have greater learning from all the efforts that have gone into making of this first edition.

Prof Shobha Tandon
Former Dean MCODS, Manipal
Karnataka, India

PREFACE

One cannot become a good cook just by watching someone else prepare a succulent meal. The modish phrase "hands on experience" describes the position very well: everyone needs direct practical involvement to become accomplished at anything. That includes the skill of writing a scientific paper. I have done my best to make this guide accessible to the students (both undergraduates and postgraduates) and faculty members of almost all the disciplines of health sciences. I wanted to help them to commit themselves to write and communicate effectively with their fellow colleagues. The book is designed specifically keeping in mind with all the core skills you need to make your mark as a high performing and an effective scientific writer. The book provides essential pointers for the beginners who are not well versed in writing a scientific paper. This compact, easy-to-use guide is a concise, yet comprehensive reference available for today's writers that guides through the step-by-step method of preparation of an article and getting it published in a good biomedical journal. It offers practical advise, clear definitions, and helpful explanations in a clear and readable style. The principles applied are applicable to all the disciplines of health sciences. This book gives clear practical advises, illustrated with examples on how to write an original research paper, a review article, case report and letter to editor.

I hope that the contents of the manual would be of value to all the scientific writers, the response be overwhelmingly positive and be most widely adopted in the nation. On the other hand, I want you to enjoy while reading the material and also attempt to write a good scientific paper which would be acceptable in an international indexed journal with high impact factor. I hope that, this book would help any trainee scientist to improve his/her skills in writing a paper and enjoy in doing so.

Dear Readers—you can now bring up your skills and give your career prospects a boost by referring *'Publish and Flourish: A Practical Guide for Effective Scientific Writing.'* I should welcome feedback on the usefulness and practicality of this first edition. Thanking you all.

Amar A Sholapurkar

ACKNOWLEDGMENTS

No book of value is written alone. Countless people helped me with this book — those who taught me and those whom I have taught. I would be adding many pages to this book if I have to name everyone to whom I am indebted. As I began to get established in my career, I quickly realized that I need to focus my mind in helping the beginners to write a scientific paper which would be publishable in good biomedical journal. My very special word of thanks to my wife who helped me initiate and focus on this problem. I would like to dedicate this edition to my parents (for their unfailing patience, belief in my abilities, constant encouragement to rise in life and who have not only stood by me but have always showered me with good wishes and blessings) and my wife (for her love, patience, and sacrificing time with me while the book was being written).

I owe an enormous debt to all the dynamic contributors for their valuable contributions. For all their many contributions, I would like to thank — Professor Wilfred CG Peh, Professor Kwan-Hoong Ng, Professor Fatema Jawad, Dr Prakash Mungli, Dr Nirmala Rao, Dr Keerthilatha M Pai, Dr KL Bairy, Dr Shailesh Lele, Dr Ranganathan Kannan, Dr Shreemathi S Mayya, Dr Kandaswamy Deivanayagam, Dr Vijay Prakash Mathur, Dr Sumanth Prasad, Dr Vidya KM and Dr Ashutosh Sharma. My special thanks to Professor Teo Eng Kiong, Editor, Singapore Medical Journal for permitting me to reproduce the materials from the articles published in Singapore Medical Journal. I would also like to thank Suzanne Paris (Rights and Permissions Coordinator, ABC-CLIO Press Santa Barbara, California, USA), Cynthia Mulrow (Senior Deputy Editor, Annals of Internal Medicine) and Dr Sivapathasundaram (Editor of Indian Journal of Dental Research) for permitting me to reproduce the materials in the book.

Closer to home, I would specially thank Professor Ramnarayan for his support, encouragement, and writing the foreword for this book. I am grateful to Professor Shobha Tandon, Dean, MCODS, Manipal for writing the foreword and for being a constant source of inspiration. I wish to express my sincere gratitude to my esteemed teacher Dr Keerthilatha M Pai, Associate Dean, Professor and Head, Department of Oral Medicine and Radiology, MCODS, Manipal for her concise and concrete suggestions as well as goodwill offered by her. I feel fortunate in having access to the resources of the Manipal University.

I extend my heartful thanks to Dr Vivekanand Kattimani (Department of Oral and Maxillofacial Surgery, Sibar Institute of Dental Sciences, Takkelapadu, Guntur) for his constant support and innovative ideas. My sincere thanks to Dr Suhas S, Professor, Department of Oral Medicine and Radiology, Siddharatha Dental College, Agalkote, Tumkur for his wonderful suggestions, honest and wise advises. I specially thank Dr Shailesh Lele, Principal, Sinhagad Dental College and Hospital, Pune for helping me in suggesting the title of the book. I would like to thank Jaypee Brothers Medical Publishers (P) Ltd, New Delhi, who helped me through the editorial process with considerable skill and caring.

Most of all, I would like to thank Almighty God for loving me so much, giving me strength and ability to achieve.

Thanking you all.

CONTENTS

Section 1
Introduction

1 Introduction

Amar A Sholapurkar

INTRODUCTION

Authors are interested in various aspects of medicine, including areas like the dentistry, allied health professions, occupational therapy, nursing, veterinary medicine, pharmacy, etc. All these areas need good writers to communicate their work effectively! The competition for tenure-track faculty positions in academia puts increasing pressure on scholars to publish new work frequently. Faculty members who focus on non-publishing-related activities (such as instructing undergraduates or postgraduates) or who publish too infrequently may find themselves out of contention for available tenure-track positions.

WHAT IS SCIENTIFIC WRITING?

If the reader is to grasp what the writer means, the writer must understand what the reader needs.

George Gopen, Judith Swan.

Humans have been able to communicate since considerable number of years, however, scientific communication is relatively rare. Science is often hard to read and write as well. The quality, clarity, understanding, communication and language of writing are the key characteristic of scientific writing which is of large and practical significance. Improving the quality of writing improves the quality of thought. Scientific writing is the basis of going to institutions, universities, libraries to gain information and knowledge and present it in a concise manner.

WHAT IS SCIENTIFIC PAPER?

The modern form of scientific publishing began in the 17th century when gentlemen decided that it would be a good idea to share the results of their endeavors among their peers, for assessment, confirmation and debate. It is very important that students, authors, researchers, editors and other concerned individuals understand what a scientific paper is. A scientific paper is a written and published report describing original research results. A well written scientific paper explains the researcher's motivation for doing/conducting a study, the study design and execution, and its eventual results. Scientific papers are written in a style that is exceedingly clear and concise. The main purpose is to inform the readers and document the approach they used to investigate that issue. Scientific paper helps to assess the observation, to repeat the experiments/study and evaluate the intellectual processes. A scientific paper usually has clear purpose, be organized systematically and target specific readers.

Scientific paper should meet the criterion of a valid publication and it should be represented clearly in component parts. It should be particularly documented in a prescribed format, i.e. IMRAD [Introduction, Methods, Results and Discussion]. The heading "Materials and Methods" is more preferred than simply "Methods". There have been different systems of organizations that were preferred by some journals. In this variation, methods appear last rather than second where we can call this as IRDAM. Whether one is writing an article about Medicine, Dentistry, Nursing, Pharmacy, etc. the IMRAD format is most preferred choice.

WHY TO WRITE A PAPER?

If I ask you a question 'why we must write' most of us would answer "to communicate", some say for "name", "fame" and others say for "promotion purpose" in their institutes and the list goes on......Yes, it is true that "communication" is very important. We write as it makes us remember, think, plan and express our thoughts. By writing we can communicate with people whom we have never met where they can judge us in the only way which is by our writing.

Preparing publishable manuscripts is an important aspect of professional life in research especially for those in academics. Scientific writing skills can be developed through long process of training and experience. Research work is incomplete unless the results are disseminated to a wider community. It is always good to make the results accessible. It gives the scientific community a good chance to find out about your work. It improves your writing skills in the sense that you will attract useful comments that you may have not thought of, which will eventually improve your future work. It is a way of paying back those who fund you. It gets you and your work well recognized in wider scientific community which is good for your career and institution. If you have a good track record of publications it becomes easier to attract funds. Publications may also lead you to be invited to peer review the work of others. You may be invited to join the editorial board of various top journals. Writing also helps you to share your discovery, your experiences with the rest of the world. If you are a junior faculty member then writing papers is fundamental to your profession and crucial to your promotion.

Research is an important tool in the discovery of new events and understanding of new phenomena. It is true that carrying a research is a challenging experience and also publishing the results is more a daunting exercise. However, carrying out research is incomplete if the results are not published. In this contest, I would like to describe a naturalist who is of no use if he is only an observer and never a writer. People who are inquisitive find the dynamic and rapidly growing field of biomedical writing that is very satisfying.

Scientific writing is an activity which all of us need to enjoy. The goal of scientific research is publications. It is a fact that authors become known by their publications. An original research, case report, review, etc. no matter how fantastic and well it is, is definitely incomplete until it is published. It is perhaps of great concern and importance that a "researcher" must provide a written document showing what was done and what was learnt from it. In short, I would like to call it as reproducibility. *A good author will not only "do" science but also "write" which can be read by the widest possible audience.*

There are three categories of people. First, are those who know the importance of writing, take trouble in doing so and will achieve in publishing their work in scientific journals. Others, who are satisfied with their writing, write without thinking about the possibility of improvement. Well the third categories are those who know that they write badly but do not worry about this and remain unsuccessful and remain unaware of their shortcoming.

Nowadays scientific publishing in peer-reviewed international indexed journals is not easy. Most of the articles (up to 30-50%) get rejected due to various reasons. Writing a paper for a scientific journal is like trying to start an old car. An inexperienced driver will obviously have problems in starting and driving a car. It is a well known fact that "difficulties in your life do not come to destroy you, but to help you realize your hidden potential" and it is my opinion that "let the difficulties know that you are difficult." This quote would be applicable in the same context where I am trying to point out the vital importance of writing a scientific paper where dedication and confidence are two qualities which you need to develop. Yes, dear young readers, you should be aware at this instance that how important, it is to get your work published in good journals to achieve the highest goals in your career.

In this book, I have tried to help the beginners through this painful period by suggesting how they can get their work published in a good scientific journal. The purpose of this book is to help undergraduates, postgraduates and the faculty of *Dental Sciences, Medical Sciences, allied health professions, occupational therapy, nursing, veterinary medicine and pharmacy* to prepare manuscripts that may be accepted for publication in high impact factor journals.

Section 2
Preliminary Considerations in Writing a Scientific Paper

2 Planning to Write a Paper

Amar A Sholapurkar

INTRODUCTION

There is an over-increasing expectation for trainees and junior doctors to publish more. It is very important to deal with some questions before you think about how to write a paper. The questions which should come to your mind are → what should you submit for publication, when should you submit and where? Satisfactory answers to these questions will save your time and will help you to write in a systematic way which will have a better chance of your article getting published in a good reputed, international indexed, peer reviewed journal.

The first step in developing a manuscript is to focus on a subject or problem that might be of significant interest to colleagues in the field. Next, the writer must conduct a detailed survey of the relevant literature, the results of which will help him or her to decide whether to actually write about the topic.

It is important that before planning to write a scientific paper certain questions regarding its worthiness, the format and target audience should be addressed. These issues are crucial and determine how well a paper is written which will eventually be acceptable for publication.

WHAT TO WRITE AND WHEN?

Successful authors combine appropriate knowledge and experience, and produce important contributions to literature. "What to write and when" is a part of planning which everyone should know. Your papers should describe or report significant experimental, theoretical or observational extensions of knowledge and practical applications of known principles in an advanced manner. In simple words write a paper which significantly adds knowledge, and understanding to the readers.

The best advise I would like to give is "Start with the Conclusion". First write down the conclusion of your study as clearly as possible. Then correlate to the hypothesis on which you are working with. Read the conclusion thrice and determine how firm the conclusions are and compare it with other articles and discuss it with your fellow colleagues or an experienced author.

Discuss carefully and note down the questions and suggestions which he/she provides. Yes, this is the time you are ready to publish. Decide whether you would like to make a long article or a short one. At this stage it is good to criticize yourself to avoid criticism from others at a later stage.

WHAT NOT TO WRITE?

The ultimate goal of a scholar article is to contribute to the advancement of knowledge, literature and its application for improving life. Unfortunately this concept is being forgotten in the research nowadays. When a paper is to be submitted for publication to any journal it is very important to establish whether the science is accurate?, is the material used in the study new and will it have any impact on clinical practice and add substantially to current knowledge? And finally, is the message appropriate for the readers?

Do not write an article simply because you think that your name will appear in print. It is my advise not to divide or cut a large article into short papers when not necessary. In case if a large study is being done and it requires many years for completion then publication of several papers may be appropriate step wise. A manuscript is worth publishing if it describes a previously unpublished work. Hence never submit an article for publication that has been already published/accepted elsewhere/the one which is being considered for publication. Do not write up the same results in different form thinking that you can publish multiple articles. This will damage your reputation. Before you write a paper, consider whether official secrecy acts from barrier to publication. You have to take legal advise for this.

WHERE TO SUBMIT A PAPER?

Before starting to write an article a provisional decision should be made about –

Which journal your article will be submitted?
Do not postpone this decision to a later stage.
Ask yourself the following questions.

- Is the topic of interest to a national or international reader?
- Is it better suited for a general or a specialist journal?
- What is the journal's impact factor (IF)? We will be discussing about impact factor in the further chapters. Greater the IF, the more widely read and cited is the journal.
- How is the general quality of the articles in that particular journal?
- What is the size of audience/readers? Usually those journals which carry advertisements have a large size of audience
- Speed of publication is also an important factor. Just observe in any article in a journal you want to publish, there will be a date of receipt of manuscript and date of acceptance for publication. Through this one can determine the exact time taken for the editorial process including the review process, proof reading, printing and binding.
- It must also be considered whether your paper is clinically based or more basic science based and send the article to that appropriate journal.
- Is the quality of photographic reproduction good?
- Point out that all journals publish a statement of the scope and purpose and accordingly one can determine if your article well suits to be submitted in that journal.
- Be careful in submitting your articles in new journals. Such journals would have low standards than the established ones. They accept almost all articles as the editor thinks it would add to his prestige or he wants to fill their pages. Such journals would not last more than a year or two. Hence avoid submitting your articles in such journals.

Determine the Prestige Factor

Yes this matters a lot. It may be that your promotions or grants will be determined based on the type of journal. It is true that a manuscript published in a prestigious journal does not equal to that published in a local nonprestigious journal. It will be more impressive to publish few articles in prestigious journals rather than publishing innumerable articles in nonprestigious journals.

Read the Instructions to Authors

The next stage would be to read the instructions to authors.

Each and every journal varies in its own style compared to others. Check whether the journal is peer reviewed and always prefer such journals. Once you have read the instructions to authors straight away start writing the manuscript in the correct format as stated in the instructions. Do not waste your time altering everything at the end. This can save a lot of time and effort.

Obtaining the Instructions to Authors

Instructions to authors will be given in all the journals. It may appear in every issue, some publish them only in the first issue of each volume and others supply on request to the editorial office. Occasionally editorial policies keep changing. As a result be sure to read the recent instructions to authors. Read it twice or thrice and then you will be in a state to decide finally whether the journal to which you are submitting is most suitable. This would be the last chance to decide whether you are submitting your article to this particular journal. You can discuss with fellow colleagues regarding the same and finally decide.

SUGGESTED READING

1. Branson RD. Anatomy of a research paper. Respir Care 2004;49(10):1222-8.
2. Brumback RA. Success at publishing in biomedical journals: hints from a journal editor. J Child Neurol 2009;24(3):370-8.
3. Deshpande SB. Art of writing a scientific paper. Indian J Physiol Pharmacol. 2006;50(1):1-6.
4. Evans M. Writing a paper. Br J Oral Maxillofac Surg 2007;45(6):485-7.
5. F. Peter Woodford. Scientific writing for graduate students. A manual on the teaching of scientific writing. 1st edn, New York: Rokefeller University press, 1968.
6. George S, Moreira K. Publishing nonresearch papers as a trainee: a recipe for beginners. Singapore Med J 2009;50(8):756-8. Review
7. Kliewer MA. Writing it up: a step-by-step guide to publication for beginning investigators. J Nucl Med Technol 2006;34(1):53-9.
8. Maeve O' Connor, F Peter Woodford. Planning. In: Maeve O' Connor, F Peter Woodford(eds). Writing Scientific Papers in English. 1st edn. England : Pitman Medical Publishing Co Ltd 1977, pp.3-6.
9. Michael Derntl. Basics of Research Paper writing and Publishing, Unpublished manuscript – Revision 2.1 – September 2009
10. Moore N. Transparency and trust: Clear definition of ghost writing would be helpful. BMJ 2004,4;329(7478):1345-6.
11. Neill US. How to write a scientific masterpiece. J Clin Invest 2007;117(12):3599-602.
12. Peh WC, Ng KH. Preparing a manuscript for submission. Singapore Med J 2009;50(8):759-61; quiz 762.
13. Provenzale JM. Ten principles to improve the likelihood of publication of a scientific manuscript. AJR Am J Roentgenol 2007;188(5):1179-82.
14. Robert A Day. Where and How to Submit the Manuscript. In:Robert A Day(ed) How to write and publish a scientific paper. 4th edn. New York: Cambridge University Press 1995, pp 90-97.
15. Robert Barrass. Scientists must Write. A guide to better writing for scientists, engineers and students. 1st edn. London: Chapman and Hall, 1978.

16. S. J. Cunningham, How to . . . write a paper, Journal of Orthodontics 2004;31:47-51.
17. Scott JT. Is it worth writing about? J R Soc Med 1993;86(1):5-6.
18. Setiati S, Harimurti K. Writing for scientific medical manuscript: a guide for preparing manuscript submitted to biomedical journals. Acta Med Indones 2007;39(1):50-5.
19. Sharp D. Kipling's guide to writing a scientific paper. Croat Med J 2002;43(3):262-7.
20. Simon RI. Authorship in forensic psychiatry: a perspective. J Am Acad Psychiatry Law 2007;35(1):18-26.
21. Temple-Smith M, Goodyear-Smith F, Gunn J. Publish or perish? Evaluation of a writing week. Aust Fam Physician 2009;38(4):257-60.

3 Deciding on Authorship
(Who Should be the Authors?)

Amar A Sholapurkar

INTRODUCTION

Now that you have read the guidelines for authors and decided that your work is ready for submitting to a suitable journal. Yes, the next step is to decide on authorship. I mean to say "whose name will appear in the manuscript and in what order". It is not at all a problem (issue) when you have worked alone where you will be the sole author in the manuscript. If at all there are multiple authors it is the best time to decide who will be the authors for the publication. This will prevent later arguments. Rational colleagues have become bitter enemies because of difference of opinions on the matter that whose names should be included in the paper and in what order.

One can define authorship as those who actively contributed to the overall design and execution of the experiments. Or in other words— Authorship credit should be given to those who

1. Substantially contribute to conception and design, acquisition of data, or analysis and interpretation of data.
2. Draft the article and revise it critically for important intellectual content and
3. Finally approve the version to be published.

The requirements for authorships are listed in the document "uniform requirements for manuscripts submitted to biomedical journals" which is compiled by the International Committee of Medical Journal Editors [ICMJE]. According to the ICMJE criteria for authorship —All the three conditions mentioned above should be met to qualify as an author. The author who is listed in the article is assumed to have made substantive intellectual contributions to the published work.

THE DONT'S OF DECIDING AN AUTHOR

- Do not include those as authors who have not contributed substantially to the published work
- Do not include as authors who simply advised you to do the work
- Do not include a person as author who gave technical assistance
- Do not include anybody as author without his/her prior intimation/approval
- Political or gift authorship should be avoided.

NUMBER OF AUTHORS

There is no hard and fast rule for the number of authors to be listed in the publication. It will usually depend on the type of manuscript whether it is a case report, short communication, letter to editor, an original research etc.

I would suggest

- Not more than 2 authors for letter to editor/short communication
- Not more than 4 authors for a case report
- Up to 6 authors for an original research paper
- Not more than 8 authors for case series
- 8 to 10 authors for a multicentric study article
- Maximum of 2 authors for a review article.

If there are more than 10 to 12 authors then this will definitely draw the attention of the editor which may require further justification. It is in the 1st authors/corresponding author's hand to keep the number of authors small.

Nowaday there is an increasing trend where the journal editors ask the authors to provide information regarding the contributions of each in the manuscript. Many journals publish this information where individual contributions to the work are mentioned. Colleagues should not ask to have their names included in the manuscript when they have not actively involved.

ORDER OF AUTHORS

The authors should normally be listed in order of importance to the work being reported. The order of authorship should be a joint decision of all the authors. The first author should be acknowledging as a senior author who is the most important one and conducted/contributed the maximum in the study. In many institutions the first author is usually the junior (eg. – postgraduate student, or a junior staff member) who has contributed the maximum in the manuscript. The other authors are listed in the descending order of contribution. If everyone has contributed equally then arrange the names alphabetically.

Some journals initially believed in listing the names in alphabetical order. Such ordering system is no longer recommended.

Editors usually do not involve in the conflicts relating to authorship issues. All the disputes among the authors should be kept private and if it is brought to editor's attention, will lead to delay in the decision of the acceptance of manuscript.

Team members who write several papers together usually have mutual understanding among themselves and take turns as being named as first author.

HOW TO LIST THE NAMES, QUALIFICATION AND ADDRESS?

For listing the name, the preferred due method is First name, Middle initial and Last name. Most journals give their qualifications after the names. Titles [Dr., Prof.] are usually not given in the literature cited. However the usage of titles depends on journal's instructions to authors. For example: Amar A Sholapurkar.

The address of the author is given where the person is working or the study conducted. If the author has changed his address before publication then the new address should be indicated in a "present address" foot note. When two or more authors are listed, each in a different institution, the address should be listed in the same order as the authors.

What is the Purpose of Providing Address?

- It serves to identify the author
- It supplies the author's mailing address. It is necessary to denote the source of reprints.

GHOST AUTHORS

A ghost author is a professional writer who is paid to write books, articles and other materials which then are officially credited to another person. Ghost authors should be distinguished from professional medical writers whose role is to assist with preparing drafts of the article with the aim of saving the author's time and effort. This service is particularly useful for authors who are not native English speakers, have language difficulties, or lack training or expertise in medical writing. The European Medical Writers Association has published guidelines to ensure that professional medical writers carry out their roles and responsibilities ethically. Professional medical writers' expertise in presenting scientific data may be beneficial in producing better quality papers.

SUGGESTED READING

1. Amacher AL. Multiauthored manuscripts. J Neurosurg 1995;82(4):700.
2. Genco RJ. Ethics in science: the publication process. Indian J Dent Res 1992;3(3):64-7.
3. Huth EJ. Responsibilities of coauthorship. Ann Intern Med 1983;99(2):256-7.
4. International Committee of Medical Journal Editors. Uniform requirements for manuscripts submitted to biomedical journals. Updated October 2008. Available at: www.icjme.org. Accessed June 14, 2010
5. Jacobs A, Wager E. European Medical Writers Association (EMWA) guidelines on the role of medical writers in developing peer-reviewed publications. Curr Med Res Opin 2005;21:317-21.
6. Lee K. Has the hunt for conflicts of interest gone too far? No. BMJ 2008; 336(7642):477.
7. Maeve O' Connor, F Peter Woodford. Preparing. In: Maeve O' Connor, F Peter Woodford(eds). Writing Scientific Papers in English. An ELSE-Ciba Foundation Guide for Authors. 1st edn. England: Pitman Medical Publishing Co Ltd; 1977. pp. 7-19.
8. Moore N. Transparency and trust: Clear definition of ghost writing would be helpful. BMJ 2004;329(7478):1345-6.
9. Novack GD. Authorship policy. Am J Ophthalmol 2009;147(1):184; author reply 184-5.
10. Peh WC, Ng KH. Authorship and acknowledgments. Singapore Med J 2009;50(6):563-5; quiz 566.
11. RD Gantra, Ethics on authorship of scientific paper, Indian Heart J 1997;49:209-11
12. Robert A Day. How to list the Authors and Addresses. In:Robert A Day(ed) How to write and publish a scientific paper. 4th edn. New York: Cambridge University Press 1995; pp. 22-8.
13. Simon RI. Authorship in forensic psychiatry: a perspective. J Am Acad Psychiatry Law 2007;35(1):18-26.
14. Sivapathasundharam B. Authorship. Indian J Dent Res 2008;19(1):1.
15. Sokol DK. The dilemma of authorship. BMJ 2008;336(7642):478.
16. Stossel TP. Has the hunt for conflicts of interest gone too far? Yes. BMJ 2008; 336(7642):476.

4 Preparing to Write a Paper

Amar A Sholapurkar

DETERMINING THE JOURNALS REQUIREMENTS

- Once you are about to start writing a paper you have to first select the journal you intend to send your article
- Once you select the journal it is important to determine if there are any special requirements of the journal. Read the instructions to author. It usually differs from journal to journal but there is no much difference. Certain journals may specify the rules of nomenclature or certain style of writing. Do it accordingly.
- If your study includes experiments on human beings or animals then ethical committee clearance is a must. You would have got the clearance before you conduct the study. Keep the certificate ready.
- Most of the journals prefer the use of international system for units of measurements [SI units]. If it specifies then use the SI units only.

COMPOSING THE WORKING TITLE AND ABSTRACT

Working Title and Abstract is a provisional or a rough version which should be prepared for the paper you intend to write. At this stage you have done the study, you know the results of which you have noted down. Hence composing the working title and abstract at this stage may not pose any difficulties. It is important to compose it as it will help you to decide what has to be included in the article and what not to be. The working title can be as long or as short as you like but it should contain the main subject of your paper which you intend to write. In your working abstract you have to be concise where you need to mention the hypothesis, method of your study, your conclusion and most importantly the significance of your study. Let the working abstract not exceed more than 5 to 6 sentences.

ORGANIZING THE PAPER [MASTER PLAN]

A scientific paper must be organized in a systematic manner. In most of the Medical/Dental/Nursing/Pharmacology journals the following format for the structure of a paper is followed.

(1) Abstract (2) Introduction (3) Materials (Subjects) and Methods (4) Results (5) Discussion and (6) Conclusions.

Read the Guidelines for authors twice or thrice or you can go through the articles of few issues of the journal to determine the structure used in that journal. Occasionally you can combine both the results and discussion.

COLLECTING THE MATERIAL

Write down all the headings, i.e. Introduction, Material(Subjects) and Methods, Results, Discussion, Conclusions.

Write all the findings related to these headings as and then when it comes to your mind. Check the laboratory findings and note it down. Add any descriptions of materials and methods or results. Do not try to assemble the items in logical order yet. Then add tables and graphs in a rough form. Write the references which are to be included in the manuscript. This is a stage where you have collected the material and compiled it but in a random manner. Anyways you have all the details pertaining to your manuscript.

DESIGNING THE TABLES AND ILLUSTRATIONS

Tables and Illustrations are the most important part of paper on which it is mostly dependent. Readers usually judge whether the text is worth reading based on the designing of the tables and illustrations. Designing will help whether you need more experiments or observations or you need to modify your conclusions. It will also help the reader to grasp the significance of tables and illustrations quickly without referring the text. It will also help to save your time in writing any unnecessary and extra words. You have to remember that tables and illustrations should convey a clear message. Keep it simpler, short and clear. Read chapters 12 and 13 for designing the tables and preparing effective illustrations respectively.

COPYRIGHT

It is not a problem if the preparations of text, tables, or illustrations are your own work. If in case you want to include such items in your manuscript from other's published or unpublished work it is mandatory to get permission from the concerned author/publisher. According to the copyright law you need to obtain a written permission from the author/publisher to reproduce the material and hence it becomes your sole responsibility to get it done before you publish.

It is not clear as to how much one can quote from someone else's work without permission but however it is said that it will be better if you get permission from the concerned author if you are quoting few lines with more than 200 words. The copyright holder may be a publisher, the author, or a third party person. If the author is not the copyright holder [owner of copyright] it is still mandatory to obtain his approval as well as from the copyright holder for the work in which the material first appeared. Copyright material should also be acknowledged.

If in case a table or illustration are taken from the original article and then modified, the permission of the copyright holder is not necessary. But a proper acknowledgment of the source from which it is picked up may be sufficient.

Occasionally tables and illustrations copied without modifications may cost some fee which the copyright holder may demand which will be anyhow stated in the copyright statement letter.

In case you want to quote some important findings from unpublished work (like those presented in conferences, lecture, meeting, or from local agencies) it is also important that you take a prior permission to do so.

Here is an example (BOX) so as to how to make a letter of permission to reproduce any material from the published work.

Box 4.1: Letter of permission to reproduce any material from the published work.

Dear Sir/Madam,

I the undersigned am planning to prepare an article titled "Efficacy of Fluconazole mouthrinse and clotrimazole mouthpaint in the treatment of oral candidiasis" I will be happy and grateful to you if you would permit me to use the following material from your published work.

I would like to use Fig 6 and Fig 7 from the article, McCullough MJ, Savage NW. Oral Candidosis and the therapeutic use of antifungal agents in dentistry. Aust Dent J 2005; 50 Suppl 2: 536 – 539. I am requesting separately to the copyright holder regarding the same.

The acknowledgments and reference to the paper will be stated in my manuscript. Please let me know if you would like to use the credit line.

Can you please sign on the agreement form and return a copy of this letter?

Thanking you.

Sincerely

Dr Amar A. Sholapurkar

I/We permit to reproduce the above specified material.

Signature

Date

Credit line to be used..

In this way type 3 copies of the letter, two of the copies need to be sent with a stamped addressed envelope, so that the copyright holder can return one signed copy and retain the other as his own record.

SUGGESTED READING

1. Bird S. Self-plagiarism, recycling fraud, and the intent to mislead. J Med Toxicol 2008;4(2):69-70.
2. Bremner J. Copyright issues: in the news again. Biomed Instrum Technol 2008;42(4):316-7.
3. Gøtzsche PC, Kassirer JP, Woolley KL, Wager E, Jacobs A, Gertel A, Hamilton C. What should be done to tackle ghostwriting in the medical literature? PLoS Med 2009;6(2):e23.
4. Johnson SH. Signing copyright transfer. Nurse Author Spring 2003;13(2):9-10.
5. Maeve O' Connor, F Peter Woodford. Preparing. In: Maeve O' Connor, F Peter Woodford(eds). Writing Scientific Papers in English. An ELSE-Ciba Foundation Guide for Authors. 1st ed. England : Pitman Medical Publishing Co Ltd; 1977. pp. 7-19.
6. Poss R, Bauer TW, Heckman JD. Copyright, ownership, and truth in data in the electronic age. J Bone Joint Surg Am 2004;86-A(4):669.
7. Robert Barrass. Scientists must Write. A guide to better writing for scientists, engineers and students. 1st edn. London: Chapman and Hall, 1978.
8. SJ Cunningham, How to . . . write a paper, Journal of Orthodontics 2004;31: 47-51
9. Walter C, Richards EP. Publish and perish. IEEE Eng Med Biol Mag 2002; 21(4):127-30,133.

Section 3
Writing a Original
Research Paper

5 Writing the First Draft–Preliminary Considerations

Amar A Sholapurkar

INTRODUCTION

Once you have finished the stage where you have prepared a rough format of the paper (you have decided on the authorship, determined the journal requirements, composed the working title and abstract, organized the paper in a proper manner, collected material, designed the tables and illustrations, and finally dealt with copyright) your manuscript is well on the road for publication. Now you need to write the text which would be quite easy if you have prepared thoroughly.

Writing the first draft will require several hours and will depend on the length of manuscript. This is a crucial time where you need to settle down in a place which will allow your remain undisturbed. Think of the article as a unit; write the first draft continuously from the beginning to end. If you know what you have to write, the article will flow best and be most coherent if it is written with one swing from the beginning to end.

THINGS TO REMEMBER WHILE YOU WRITE THE FIRST DRAFT

- Collect the material you have prepared and start writing or type the first draft
- If the paper is short then try to finish writing in one sitting
- At this stage do not worry about the style or grammar
- No matter what style the journal uses for citing the references in the text, use the name – and – date system [Witkop et al; 1982] in writing the draft. If the journal uses numbering system then change the names to numbers after the preparation of final draft
- Try to use appropriate tense and verbs in writing the first draft. Past tense is usually used for observations, and conclusions
- Find out as much as you can from the literature and then match your style of writing accordingly

- Every word or phrase should be appropriate and each sentence should convey a whole thought
- Convey your thoughts clearly and accurately
- If you know what you wish to communicate but have difficulty in getting started then look at the opening sentences of similar articles by other authors. The only rule about beginning is to come straight to the point
- Length of sentence is also important in preparing the first draft. Long sentences may indicate that you have not thought about what you wish to say. Hence revise any long sentence if it is difficult to read or, make it into two or three shorter sentences. However long sentences if properly constructed may be easier to read and carry more weightage than those with shorter sentences
- Some authors consider that style of writing is not important. But it is not so practically. It is said that the secret in style of writing is to have something to say as clearly as you can. Good style depends upon your intelligence, imagination, good taste, careful planning and your attention towards scientific writing.

6) *Preparing the Title*

Amar A Sholapurkar

INTRODUCTION

The title is the first and most important part of an article. Just as we read quickly through the headlines of newspaper every morning to see if there is anything worth reading that day, we tend to read the title first and if one feels it to relevant and catchy, we proceed reading the rest of the matter. Similarly readers read the contents page of the journal. On reading the title, they decide whether the topic is worth reading and then look at the Abstract and Introduction. Hence it is important that the title should be appropriate and attract the attention of the readers.

Title is one which is read by thousands of people. Many people will read the title either in the original journal or in abstracting and indexing where you call it as secondary publication. Title is considered as a signport that tells the reader about your paper and diverts their attention and creates interest and curiosity in reading your paper.

I would repeat again that title of a paper is the one which is read most and usually the first. The electronic indexing services rely heavily on the accuracy of the title to allow users to find papers relevant to their queries. If the title is unable to attract the attention of the potential reader, the rest of the article is less likely to be read. Housing a good title is therefore desirable.

HOW SHOULD BE A GOOD TITLE?

"Day" defines a good title "as the fewest possible words that adequately describe the contents of the paper.

The following are the requirements of a good title.
- Length of title—Ideally speaking long titles are often meaningless than shorter ones. Usually long titles contain waste words. On the

other hand, titles which are too short often use words which are too general. Examples of waste words → A, An, the, such words are useless for indexing purposes

- Titles must be functional, should be direct, and need not be dull
- Title should give a clear indication of the subject and scope of the work
- Some journals print list of keywords and hence keywords should be included in the title as much as possible
- Always start the title with an important word
- Title should be unambiguous
- Authors should avoid the temptation of adding extraneous details such as the objectives, methods or results from the study
- Indexing and abstracting services depend heavily on the accuracy of titles. Improperly titled articles may not reach the intended audience. Hence, the title should also ideally contain the keywords of the subject matter
- Use simple language
- Be concise, memorable, informative and descriptive
- Be careful of syntax (word order). Most of the grammatical errors in titles are due to faulty word order
- Titles should never contain abbreviations.

What is a "Running title"?

Some journals require a running title which is a short version of the title. This is usually printed as a header at the top of each or alternate journal page. The running title is limited in length by a maximum number of characters specified in the journals author guidelines. It is wise to suggest an appropriate running title on the title page of the manuscript.

SUGGESTED READING

1. Basmajian JV. Quality in Scientific Writing. Can Med Assoc J 1964;90:1121-5.
2. Branson RD. Anatomy of a research paper. Respir Care 2004;49(10):1222-8.
3. Brumback RA. Success at publishing in biomedical journals: hints from a journal editor. J Child Neurol 2009;24(3):370-8.
4. Deshpande SB. Art of writing a scientific paper. Indian J Physiol Pharmacol 2006;50(1):1-6.
5. Evans M Writing a paper. Br J Oral Maxillofac Surg 2007;45(6):485-7.
6. F. Peter Woodford. Scientific writing for graduate students. A manual on the teaching of scientific writing. 1st edn, New York: Rokefeller University press, 1968.

7. Fiona Moss. Titles, abstracts and authors. In: George M Hall(ed). How to write a Paper. 3rd edn. Noida, India; Byword Viva Publishers Private Limited; 2004. pp. 42-50.
8. Kliewer MA. Writing it up: a step-by-step guide to publication for beginning investigators. AJR Am J Roentgenol 2005;185(3):591-6.
9. Kliewer MA. Writing it up: a step-by-step guide to publication for beginning investigators. J Nucl Med Technol 2006;34(1):53-9.
10. Michael Derntl. Basics of Research Paper writing and Publishing, Unpublished manuscript – Revision 2.1 – September 2009
11. Neill US. How to write a scientific masterpiece. J Clin Invest 2007;117(12):3599-602.
12. Peh WC, Ng KH. Title and title page. Singapore Med J 2008;49(8):607-8; quiz 609.
13. Provenzale JM. Ten principles to improve the likelihood of publication of a scientific manuscript. AJR Am J Roentgenol 2007;188(5):1179-82.
14. Robert A Day. How to prepare the Title. In:Robert A Day(ed) How to write and publish a scientific paper. 4th ed. New York: Cambridge University Press; 1995. pp. 15-21.
15. Robert Barrass. Scientists must Write. A guide to better writing for scientists, engineers and students. 1st edn. London: Chapman and Hall, 1978.
16. S. J. Cunningham, How to . . . write a paper, Journal of Orthodontics 2004;47-51.
17. Setiati S, Harimurti K. Writing for scientific medical manuscript: a guide for preparing manuscript submitted to biomedical journals. Acta Med Indones 2007;39(1):50-5.
18. Sharp D. Kipling's guide to writing a scientific paper. Croat Med J 2002; 43(3):262-7.
19. Szklo M. Quality of scientific articles. Rev Saude Publica 2006;40 Spec no: 30-5.
20. Temple-Smith M, Goodyear-Smith F, Gunn J. Publish or perish? Evaluation of a writing week. Aust Fam Physician 2009;38(4):257-60.
21. Van Way CW 3rd. Writing a scientific paper. Nutr Clin Pract. 2007;22(6):636-40. Review.

7 Preparing the Abstract

Amar A Sholapurkar

INTRODUCTION

Having read your title, the reader will next want to know more information without having gone through the whole long article to get the "meat". This is the purpose of an abstract. In short an abstract is a succinct (one paragraph) summary of the entire manuscript. Although it is located at the beginning of the paper, it is the easiest to write.

An abstract is often the only part of the manuscript that is read by most of the readers. Hence, it should be written in such a way that it encourages the potential readers to read the whole paper. Basically an abstract comprises of a one paragraph summary of the whole paper. They have become very important as electronic publication databases are the primary means of finding research reports in the subject area of concern.

FEATURES OF ABSTRACT

The following are the features of abstract.
- It puts your work into context and presents your conclusions
- It tells what you have done and what you found out
- It does not include statistics
- It clearly states the implications of your findings
- They are usually short and mostly do not exceed 250 words in most of the journals. It should be noted that if the abstract of a scientific paper is more than 250 words then MEDLINE just cuts it off after the 250th word which will make it an incomplete abstract
- There are no abbreviations or acronyms and usually have no redundant information
- There are no illustrative elements like tables and figures
- It does not include references.

Abstracts may be classified as informative, descriptive (indicative), or a mixture of both.

Informative abstract are best for papers describing original research. Hence write informative abstract wherever possible. It is designed to condense the paper and briefly state the problem, method used in the study and the principal data and conclusions.

Indicative (Descriptive) abstract is used for review papers, conference reports etc. It omits all the numerical data.

WHAT IS STRUCTURED ABSTRACT AND UNSTRUCTURED ABSTRACT?

Structured Abstract

Many journals suggest the use of structured abstracts. Such abstracts are usually applicable for research articles. It follows the following headings → (1) background (2) Objective (3) Methods (4) Results and (5) Conclusions. This corresponds to 4 sections of the paper. Introduction, Materials and Methods, Results and discussion. Even if the journal does not specify structured abstract, it is wise and useful way of writing an abstract as it is easy for the readers to understand and see your findings.

To write the abstract, just go through the paper. Each heading in the abstract should be no more than three sentences so that there is no need to elaborate it.

- Introduction section—It is also called as Background section in some journals. It should contain the statement of hypothesis
- Objective—State the objectives of the study in an impressive style
- Methods—Methods should detail the study design in short and outline the procedures and variables
- Results should not include unnecessary points but report only principal findings
- Conclusion should summarize the interpretation of the results and state whether the hypothesis was supported or rejected. It should be limited to one or two sentences. There should be direct correlation between the purpose of the study and the conclusions.

Note: The abstract is usually written after all the basic components of the paper have been written. Write the abstract in the past tense because it refers to the work done. Nothing can be included in the abstract that does not appear in the body of the paper.

Unstructured Abstracts

Unstructured abstracts become standard for reviews, case reports etc.
* Use each and every word carefully. If you can write the abstract in 150 words then do not use 250 words unnecessarily.

SUMMARY

In short an abstract is a summary of the entire manuscript. As stated earlier, an abstract is often the only part of the manuscript that is read by most of the readers and hence, it should be written in such a way that it encourages the potential readers to read the whole paper.

SUGGESTED READING

1. Branson RD. Anatomy of a research paper. Respir Care 2004;49(10):1222-8.
2. Brumback RA. Success at publishing in biomedical journals: hints from a journal editor. J Child Neurol 2009;24(3):370-8.
3. Deshpande SB. Art of writing a scientific paper. Indian J Physiol Pharmacol 2006;50(1):1-6
4. Evans M. Writing a paper. Br J Oral Maxillofac Surg 2007;45(6):485-7.
5. F. Peter Woodford. Scientific writing for graduate students. A manual on the teaching of scientific writing. 1st edn, New York: Rokefeller University press; 1968.
6. Fiona Moss. Titles, abstracts and authors. In: George M Hall(ed). How to write a Paper. 3rd edn. Noida, India; Byword Viva Publishers Private Limited; 2004. pp. 42-50.
7. Kliewer MA. Writing it up: a step-by-step guide to publication for beginning investigators. AJR Am J Roentgenol 2005;185(3):591-6.
8. Kliewer MA. Writing it up: a step-by-step guide to publication for beginning investigators. J Nucl Med Technol 2006;34(1):53-9.
9. Maeve O' Connor, F Peter Woodford. Refining. In: Maeve O' Connor, F Peter Woodford(eds). Writing Scientific Papers in English. An ELSE-Ciba Foundation Guide for Authors. 1st edn. England: Pitman Medical Publishing Co Ltd; 1977. pp. 46-58.
10. Michael Derntl. Basics of Research Paper writing and Publishing, Unpublished manuscript – Revision 2.1 – September 2009
11. Neill US. How to write a scientific masterpiece. J Clin Invest 2007;117(12):3599-602.
12. Peh WC, Ng KH. Abstract and keywords. Singapore Med J 2008;49(9):664-5.
13. Provenzale JM. Ten principles to improve the likelihood of publication of a scientific manuscript. AJR Am J Roentgenol 2007;188(5):1179-82.
14. Robert A Day. How to prepare the Abstract. In:Robert A Day(ed) How to write and publish a scientific paper. 4th ed. New York: Cambridge University Press; 1995.29-32.
15. S J Cunningham, How to . . . write a paper, Journal of Orthodontics 2004;31:47-51.
16. Setiati S, Harimurti K. Writing for scientific medical manuscript: a guide for preparing manuscript submitted to biomedical journals. Acta Med Indones 2007;39(1):50-5.

17. Sharp D. Kipling's guide to writing a scientific paper. Croat Med J 2002;43(3):262-7.
18. Szklo M. Quality of scientific articles. Rev Saude Publica 2006;40 Spec no: 30-5.
19. Temple-Smith M, Goodyear-Smith F, Gunn J. Publish or perish? Evaluation of a writing week. Aust Fam Physician 2009;38(4):257-60.
20. Van Way CW 3rd. Writing a scientific paper. Nutr Clin Pract 2007;22(6): 636-40.

8 Writing the Keywords

Amar A Sholapurkar

Keywords are the one that people use when searching for articles in literature indexes. They are usually 3 to 10 words or concise—phrase that may reveal the main topic of the study and is usually stated along with the abstract. These will help the indexers in cross-indexing the article. A proper keyword will help the paper to be located easily during a literature search, particularly an online search. Choosing a keyword is very important and for that the authors should understand the subject and purpose of the study. The most important concepts should be selected and then they should be expressed in words. The keywords cannot be picked up simply by the authors. They must appear in the National Library of Medicines List of Medical Subject headings (MeSH) at http://www.nLm.nih.gov/mesh/MBrowser.htmL. MeSH is the US National Library of Medicine(NLM) controlled vocabulary thesaurus and is used for indexing articles from 4800 of the world's leading biomedical journals for the MEDLINE/PubMed database. MeSH descriptors are arranged in both an alphabetical and a hierarchical structure.

SUGGESTED READING

1. Branson RD. Anatomy of a research paper. Respir Care 2004;49(10):1222-8.
2. Brumback RA. Success at publishing in biomedical journals: hints from a journal editor. J Child Neurol 2009;24(3):370-8.
3. Deshpande SB. Art of writing a scientific paper. Indian J Physiol Pharmacol 2006;50(1):1-6.
4. Evans M. Writing a paper. Br J Oral Maxillofac Surg 2007;45(6):485-7.
5. Kliewer MA. Writing it up: a step-by-step guide to publication for beginning investigators. AJR Am J Roentgenol 2005;185(3):591-6.
6. Kliewer MA. Writing it up: a step-by-step guide to publication for beginning investigators. J Nucl Med Technol 2006;34(1):53-9.
7. Michael Derntl. Basics of Research Paper writing and Publishing, Unpublished manuscript – Revision 2.1 – September 2009.

8. Neill US. How to write a scientific masterpiece. J Clin Invest 2007;117(12):3599-602.
9. Peh WC, Ng KH. Abstract and keywords. Singapore Med J 2008;49(9):664-5; quiz 666.
10. Provenzale JM. Ten principles to improve the likelihood of publication of a scientific manuscript. AJR Am J Roentgenol 2007;188(5):1179-82.
11. S. J. Cunningham, How to . . . write a paper, Journal of Orthodontics 2004;31:47-51.
12. Setiati S, Harimurti K. Writing for scientific medical manuscript: a guide for preparing manuscript submitted to biomedical journals. Acta Med Indones 2007;39(1):50-5.
13. Sharp D. Kipling's guide to writing a scientific paper. Croat Med J 2002;43(3):262-7.
14. Temple-Smith M, Goodyear-Smith F, Gunn J. Publish or perish? Evaluation of a writing week. Aust Fam Physician 2009;38(4):257-60.

9 Writing the Introduction

Amar A Sholapurkar

INTRODUCTION

The introduction section is normally placed in the beginning of text proper after the abstract. The introduction is what motivates the readers to read a paper. In some journals the introduction section is also called as "Background". The introduction should allow the reader to understand the rest of the paper without referring to previous publication on the topic. It is the first component of IMRAD structure of an original article. Introducing a scientific paper is same as introducing a person to a group of individuals. One often introduces a person by his name, followed by status, place of origin, his/her achievements etc. On the other hand, in a paper, one speaks of the background of the theme of work that is being reported, like what other workers have done so far and what has to be done in future.

TIPS TO WRITE AN INTRODUCTION

The question "Why did you start the study?" is usually answered by Introduction. Following are few tips so as to how an introduction is written ideally.

- It should be simple, brief and straight forward
- It should not contain unnecessary information which distracts or mislead the reader from the main message
- It should not contain discussion, review of literature, materials and methods and conclusions
- Do not give extensive criticism on other's work
- Few references may be quoted in the introduction. It is a bad practice to quote many references. Instead refer the article which gives many references (usually a review article) and quote it
- It should include the key papers in the field of research

- The introduction section is usually longest for original articles and shortest for case reports
- The purpose of the introduction is providing a rationale for the study information and purpose
- An ideal introduction should be of 2 to 3 paragraph.

The *first paragraph* describes the natured problem or issue, i.e. what is the problem? You should pick-up some or most words from the title. It usually provides background information by quoting few references. This background information should include a brief summary of what has already been done. Do not miss out any important reference. Start the background information initially with general facts and then moving to more specific facts related to the study.

The *second paragraph* should elaborate on the importance of the problem [Or motivation for current investigation] and list the unresolved issues [Why your paper is needed?]. In other words, state whether the study you are conducting is the next step of the previous studies OR you are conducting a study because prior studies have been somehow deficient in some way. If the purpose of conducting your study is the former one, then literature review should focus on most important 2 to 4 articles and show how this study would be the next step. If the purpose of your study is the later one then 2 to 4 references should be cited and their deficiencies stated.

The *third paragraph* should describe the rationale (reason/purpose) of the current study and contain the research question and the hypothesis and state, how it relates to previous work. The author should provide the information about how the hypothesis for the study or idea came about, either from his/her personal thoughts and experiences or from referenced work by others. Remember that neither the editors, reviewers nor the readers are interested to read the studies which are repetition of what has been done previously by others. The last sentence of this paragraph should begin with "The purpose of this study was to" ....

SUMMARY

Introduction is the first component of IMRAD structure of an original article. The question "Why did you start the study?" is usually answered by Introduction. In short, the introduction should allow the reader to understand the rest of the paper without referring to previous publication on the topic.

SUGGESTED READING

1. Branson RD. Anatomy of a research paper. Respir Care 2004;49(10):1222-8.
2. Brumback RA. Success at publishing in biomedical journals: hints from a journal editor. J Child Neurol 2009;24(3):370-8.
3. Deshpande SB. Art of writing a scientific paper. Indian J Physiol Pharmacol 2006;50(1):1-6.
4. Evans M. Writing a paper. Br J Oral Maxillofac Surg 2007;45(6):485-7.
5. F. Peter Woodford. Scientific writing for graduate students. A manual on the teaching of scientific writing. 1st edn, New York: Rokefeller University press, 1968.
6. Kliewer MA. Writing it up: a step-by-step guide to publication for beginning investigators. AJR Am J Roentgenol 2005;185(3):591-6.
7. Kliewer MA. Writing it up: a step-by-step guide to publication for beginning investigators. J Nucl Med Technol 2006;34(1):53-9.
8. Michael Derntl. Basics of Research Paper writing and Publishing, Unpublished manuscript – Revision 2.1 – September 2009
9. Naik SR, Aggarwal R. 'Introduction' and 'discussion' in a scientific paper. J Assoc Physicians India 1991;39(9):703-4.
10. Neill US. How to write a scientific masterpiece. J Clin Invest 2007;117(12):3599-602.
11. Peh WC, Ng KH. Writing the introduction. Singapore Med J 2008;49(10):756-7; quiz758.
12. Provenzale JM. Ten principles to improve the likelihood of publication of a scientific manuscript. AJR Am J Roentgenol 2007;188(5):1179-82.
13. Richard Smith. Introductions. In: George M Hall(ed). How to write a Paper. 3rd edn. Noida, India; Byword Viva Publishers Private Limited 2004;pp.6-15.
14. Robert A Day. How to Write the Introduction. In:Robert A Day(ed) How to write and publish a scientific paper. 4th edn. New York: Cambridge University Press 1995;33-5.
15. Setiati S, Harimurti K. Writing for scientific medical manuscript: a guide for preparing manuscript submitted to biomedical journals. Acta Med Indones 2007;39(1):50-5.
16. Sharp D. Kipling's guide to writing a scientific paper. Croat Med J 2002; 43(3):262-7.
17. Szklo M. Quality of scientific articles. Rev Saude Publica 2006;40:30-5.
18. Temple-Smith M, Goodyear-Smith F, Gunn J. Publish or perish. Evaluation of a writing week. Aust Fam Physician 2009;38(4):257-60.

10 Describing How to Write the Materials and Methods

Wilfred CG Peh and Kwan-Hoong Ng

INTRODUCTION

The "materials and methods" section of a scientific paper is the second component of the conventional IMRAD (Introduction, Materials and methods, Results and Discussion) structure of an original article. However, minor variations often exist among different journals; and this section may also be known by other names such as Subjects and Methods, Patients and Methods, Methodology, or simply, Methods. Authors should always check the individual journal's "Instructions to Authors" or "Author Guidelines" for details of in house style requirements.

The "materials and methods" section is probably the most important part of a manuscript, as fundamental flaws in this section will invariably lead to rejection during the peer review process. The main purpose of the "materials and methods" section is to describe the study in sufficient detail such that other competent researchers are able to repeat the study, based on their reading of this section. The components of the "materials and methods" section should address the following questions:

- What was done?
- How was it done?
- How will the data be analyzed?
- Which type of study, location of study and period and duration of study?

Ideally, the "materials and methods" section should be written before the start of the study, i.e. during the planning stage. It makes sense for the author and research team to refine and perfect the way the study should be conducted before embarking on it as good research should be well justified, well planned and appropriately designed enough to address the research question. It is also recommended that the input of a biostatistician be sought during this study design stage, so that statistical issues, including power calculations, are resolved prior to the start of the research. A prestudy "materials and methods" section may also be part of a grant proposal.

When the study has been completed, the "materials and methods" is usually the first section to be written during manuscript preparation. The way the study was actually done, starting with the research plan, how the subjects were recruited (or how the materials were obtained), and the various methods used to obtain the data should be described in chronological order. The findings for all the items included in this section should also subsequently appear in the results section. Passive voice and third person in the past tense is recommended for writing this section.

MATERIALS

How were the subjects recruited? Were they recruited prospectively or collected retrospectively? (Example 1). The subjects should include patients, normal volunteers or animals, as well as controls. The source population should be defined, and the sampling method used described in detail. Both the inclusion and exclusion criteria used for recruitment of the study group should be clearly stated (Example 2). For selection of the control group, how they relate to the study group should be described, e.g. matched by age, gender, ethnicity, clinical condition (Example 3). Details are important. For animal subjects, details such as genus, species and strain; age, gender, nutritional state; physiological or pathological status (e.g. pregnant, castration); rearing method; diet (e.g. constituents and sources) and name of supplier are expected (Example 4).

Medical research involving human studies should be performed according to principles outlined in the World Medical Association Declaration of Helsinki (59th WMA General Assembly, Seoul, 2008). Approval from a formally-constituted review board (Institutional review board [IRB] or ethics committee) is required for all studies involving humans, medical records, and human tissues. Informed consent from participants of the study should always be sought; if this is not possible, the IRB should decide whether this is ethically acceptable (Example 5). The IRB may also waive the requirement for informed consent, particularly for retrospective studies or case record reviews. Animal experiments require compliance with ethical and existing regulatory principles, and local licensing arrangements and guidelines. Statements indicating approval from the IRB, institutional animal care committee or other appropriate bodies; and whether or informed consent was obtained or waived, should be provided.

METHODS

As reproducibility of the study methodology is vital, complete details of new or modified methods, precision of measurements and statistical analysis should be provided. For apparatus or equipment, model details, manufacturer and city of manufacture should be stated (Example 6). Any modifications made to equipment or construction of new equipment should be described, and if necessary, illustrated by photographs or diagrams. For drugs or chemicals, the exact dosages, route of administration, generic name, supplier's name, and chemical name for non-standard drugs, should be provided. The exact types, sources and supplier's name should be provided for tissues, tissue cultures, cell lines, immune sera, bacterial cultures and viruses, culture media and buffers, and reagents (Example 7).

The evaluation methods used should be comprehensively described, e.g. number of observers, whether they were blinded or not, whether assessments were done independently or by consensus, and if done, the exact time period between readings (Example 8). Was the evaluation prospectively or retrospectively performed? Was a grading system used? Were evaluations recorded on specially-designed forms? If so, all the items should be listed and if relevant, this form may need to be included as an appendix. Intra- and inter-observation variations may need to be calculated.

The method of proof should be clearly stated. This includes surgery, biopsy, histology (Example 9) and other established methods such as blood and specimen cultures, and biochemical tests (Example 10). Absence of disease on follow-up and the duration of follow-up should also be documented, if relevant.

STATISTICAL EVALUATION

Which test was used, why was particular test chosen, on what data, to determine what? Enough detail should be provided so that results can be independently verified. Ideally, standard statistical methods should be used. For standard tests, provide name, version, company, and city (Example 11). If not well known, the test should be described in detail. For advanced or unusual tests, a reference should be provided. It is good practice to again seek the advice of a biostatistician during manuscript preparation.

COMMON PROBLEMS

- Insufficient details of methodology, i.e. not specific and not comprehensive
- Misplaced information, e.g. results appearing in the "materials and methods" section, and vice-versa
- Wrong statistical test used
- Providing irrelevant information
- Noncompliance with journal's "instructions to authors".

SUMMARY

The "materials and methods" section should state clearly how the study was done, how the data was collected and how it was analyzed. Above all, reproducibility is the key. To achieve this, this section should contain sufficient detailed information to enable any researcher to replicate the study.

EXAMPLES

Example 1: Retrospective study showing how subjects were recruited*

This was a retrospective study consisting of 400 patients who had undergone an appendicectomy between October 2006 and May 2008 and who were identified from the operation note database of the Department of Surgery, Raja Isteri Pengiran Anak Saleha (RIPAS) Hospital, Brunei Darussalem.

Example 2: Definitions of inclusion and exclusion criteria**

The inclusion criteria were infants with respiratory distress, an oxygen index (OI) ≥ 25 despite HFOV support (Sensormedic high frequency oscillator. 3100A. Yorba. Linda, CA. USA) and echocardiographic evidence of PPHN. The echocardiographic features of PPHN were a

---

Reproduced with permission from: Chong CF, Adi MIW, Thien A, et al. Development of the RIPASA score: a new appendicitis scoring system for the diagnosis of acute appendicitis. Singapore Med J 2010; 51(3):220-5.

**Reproduced with permission from: Boo NY, Rohana J, Yong SC, et al. Inhaled nitric oxide and intravenous magnesium sulphate for the treatment of persistent pulmonary hypertension of the newborn. Singapore Med J 2010;51(2):144-50.*

normal cardiac anatomy with right-to-left shunt at the foramen ovale and/or ductus arteriosus, with or without dilatation of the right ventricle. The exclusion criteria were infants with lethal congenital anomalies (except congenital diaphragmatic hernia), substantial bleeding diathesis (e.g. massive intracranial hemorrhage, intraventricular hemorrhage $\geq$ Grade 3, platelet count < 50,000/L), active seizures, blood pressure that could not be stabilized, or gestational age ·< 34 weeks.

Example 3: Selection of control and study groups*

The rats were randomized and divided into four groups. Groups 1 and 2, the control groups, comprising six young rats and six adult rats, respectively, were injected with saline. Groups 3 and 4, the injury groups, also comprising six young rats and six adult rats, respectively, were injected with $FeCl_3$. All the rats were observed for six hours post-injection for seizure events, after which they were killed and decapitated. Their left hemispheres were extirpated and tested for the MDA levels and SOD activities.

Example 4: Details of animal subjects, including ethical approval **

Adult male Wistar rats whose body weight ranged from 150 to 160 g were obtained from the Central Animal House, Rajah Muthiah Medical College and Hospital, Annamalai University, India. They were housed in an environmentally controlled room that was maintained at a temperature of 22°C ± 2°C and humidity 55% ± 5, with a 12-hour light/dark cycle. The animals received a standard pellet diet (Karnataka State Agro Corporation. Bangalore, India) and tap water ad libitu. They were cared for according to the principles and guidelines of the Institutional Ethical Committee of Animal Care, Rajah Muthiah Medical College and Hospital, Annamalai University, and all treatment procedures were approved by the Committee.

Reproduced with permission from: Golden N, Darmadipura S, Bagiada NA. The difference in seizure incidences between young and adult rats related to lipid peroxidation after intracortical injection of ferric chloride. Singapore Med J 2010;51(2):105-9.

** Reproduced with permission from: Pooranaperundevi M, Sumiyabanu MS, Viswanathan P, et al. Insulin resistance induced by a high-fructose diet potentiates thioacetamide hepatotoxicity. Singapore Med J 2010;51(5):389-98.*

Example 5: Ethical approval and informed consent from parents*

This was a randomized controlled trial carried out at the neonatal intensive care unit of the Hospital Universiti Kebangsaan Malaysia over a 37-month period, between 1 April, 2000 and 30 April, 2003. The study protocol was approved by the hospital scientific and ethics committees. Written parental informed consent was obtained before randomization.

Example 6: Details of equipment used**

All CTPA examinations were performed with multi-detector scanners using a standard protocol. The CT machines were either Somaton Sensation 16 or Somaton Sensation 64 (Siemens, Erlangen, Germany). Intravenous iodinated contrast agent (Omnipaque 350) was delivered at a rate of 3 ml/sec via mechanical injectors, either Stellant (Medrad, PA, USA) or Dual Shot (Nemoto, Japan). A total of 90 ml of contrast was administered.

Example 7: Details of fluorescence *in situ* hybridization (FISH) analysis***

FISH was performed on touch imprints from fresh tumor samples and fixed immediately in modified Carnoy's fixative (3: 1 methanol/glacial acetic acid). Hybridization and wash protocols were performed as described elsewhere. The slides were counterstained with 4'6-diamidino-2-phenylindole (DAPI) in antifade solution (Vectorshield, Vector Laboratories, Burlingame, CA, USA). The FISH preparations were analyzed under an Olympus BX 60 fluorescence microscope equipped with filter sets for DAPI, FITC, rhodamine, dual band-pass for FITC/rhodamine and tripe band- pass for FITC/rhodamine/DAPI. Images were acquired via a CCD camera (COHU) and digitized and processed with Powergene MacProbe Imaging software (Applied

---

* *Reproduced with permission from: Boo NY, Rohana J, Yong SC, et al. Inhaled nitric oxide and intravenous magnesium sulphate for the treatment of persistent pulmonary hypertension of the newborn. Singapore Med J 2010;51(2):144-50.*

** *Reproduced with permission from: Eng CW, Wansaicheong G, Goh SKJ, et al. Exclusion of acute pulmonary embolism: computed tomography pulmonary angiogram or D-dimer? Singapore Med J 2009;50(4):403-6.*

*** *Reproduced with permission from: Yong MH, Hwang WS, Knight LA, et al. Comparing histopathological classifiation with MYCN, Ip36 and 17q status detected by fluorescence in situ hybridization from 14 untresated primary neuroblastomas in Singapore. Singapore Med J 2009;50(11):1090-4.*

Imaging, Newcastle-upon-Tyne, UK; now Genetix Ltd). At least 100 interphase cells were scored for MYCN status and 50 to 200 cells were scored for 1p and 17q statuses. For one case (Patient 10), 1p deletion and 17q gain studies by FISH were not performed because of insufficient cells and a severely crushed tumor.

Example 8: Evaluation of ultrasonographical images and evaluation criteria*

AU subjects underwent ultrasonographical examination of the gall bladder and common bileduct during the study period. The SCI patients were examined 108 ± 25 days after the trauma and all cases within the six months from the injury onset. Ultrasonographical examinations were performed using two echo units (HDI 5000 and HDI 3500, ATL Ultrasound Inc, Bothell, WA, USA) equipped with a high-resolution 2 to 5 MHz curved transducer. The examinations were carried out by three independent experienced radiologists blinded to the patients' identities, and the images were interpreted in consensus. For each ultrasonographical session, the transducer was placed over the right upper abdominal quadrant. Biliary sludge was defined as non-shadowing low-amplitude echoes layering in the dependent portion of the gallbladder or common bileduct and forming a fluid-fluid level with changes in the patient position. Gallstones were defined as echogenic intraluminal filling defects of the gallbladder or common bileduct with an accompanying posterior acoustic shadow, moving freely with gravity. In cases of lithiasis, the size of the gallstones was measured. The gallbladder wall thickness and echogenicity, as well as the bile duct width were registered in all subjects.

Example 9: Proof of diagnosis by histological criteria**

For the diagnosis of FA, colloid-filled follicles having uniform-appearing epithelial cells together with a well-confined capsule formation were identified. Careful observations to exclude malignancy and to differentiate from NG were performed. In HA, the lesions composed of

---

* *Reproduced with permission from: Baltas CS, Balanika AP, Sgantzos MN, et al. Gallstones and biliary sludge in Greek patients with complete high spinal cord injury: an ultrasonographical evaluation. Singapore Med J 2009; 50(9):889-93.*

** *Reproduced with permission from: Htwe TT, Hamdi MM, Swethadri GK, et al. Incidence of thyroid malignancy among goitrous thyroid lesions from the Sarawak General Hospital 2000-2004. Singapore Med J 2009; 50(7):724-8.*

cells with abundant eosinophilic cytoplasm and small regular nuclei were taken into account. For NG, thyroid nodules containing colloid-rich follicles lined by flattened, inactive epithelium were noted. TG was diagnosed by the presence of crowded glands and follicles lined by tall columnar epithelia. The enlarged epithelial cells project into the lumens of the follicles and the scalloped appearance of the edges of the colloid are diagnostic. In HT, the thyroid parenchymas with a dense active lymphocytic infiltration are diagnostic.

Example 10: Proof of diagnosis using biochemical criteria*

The diagnosis of adrenal insufficiency was made using the following criteria: baseline cortisol levels of < 550 nmol/L: cortisol response following LDT, increment of cortisol < 250 nmol/L and peak cortisol <700 nmol/L; and following SDT, increment of cortisol < 250 nmol/L [18] and peak cortisol < 938 nmol/L. Statistical analysis was performed using the Wilcoxon rank test for repeated measurements. The Mann-Whitney test was used to determine the significance between two groups (survival and nonsurvival) and for numerical variables. A p-value of < 0.05 was deemed to be of statistical significance.

Example 11: Description of statistical tests**

Statistical analysis was performed using the Statistical Package for the Social Sciences 13.0 version for Windows program (SPSS Inc, Chicago, IL, USA). The continuous variables are described as average ± standard deviation and median, interquartile range. The categorical variables were presented in terms of their frequency. For a comparison of the means with a normal distribution between the patient groups, student's t-test and one-way ANO/VA were used as parametric tests. For a comparison of the means without a normal distribution between the patient groups, Mann-Whitney U-test and Kruskal-Wallis test were used as nonparametric tests. The presence of differences was tested using the Mann-Whitney U-test, and the source of the difference was found

---

* *Reproduced with permission from: Norasyikin AW, Norlela S, Rozita H, et al. Adrenal insufficiency in acute coronary syndrome. Singapore Med J 2009;50(10):962-6.*

** *Reproduced from: Ozturk A, Ozkan Y, Akgoz S, et al. The risk factors for mortality in elderly patients with hip fractures: postoperative one-year results. Singapore Med J 2010; 51(2):137-43.*

with the Kruskal-Wallis test. In order to compare the categorical variables between the patient groups, Pearson's chi-square, Fisher's exact, Kolmogorov-Smirnov and Mantel-Haenszel chi-square tests were used. After the normality assumptions were assessed, a two-way mixed design ANOVA (with independent measures on mortality) was performed with the Greenhouse-Geisser adjustment. The relationships between patient characteristics and survival were analzed by the Kaplan-Meier and Cox Regression Analyses (Forward LR). A p-value of less than 0.05 was regarded as significant.

SUGGESTED READING

1. International Committee of Medical Journal Editors. Uniform requirements for manuscripts submitted to biomedical journals: writing and editing for biomedical publications. Updated October 2008. Available at: www.icmje.org.
2. Ng KH, Peh WCG. Writing the materials and methods. Singapore Med J 2008; 49:856-9.
3. Peh WCG, Ng KH. Basic structure and types of scientific papers. Singapore Med J 2008;49:522-5.
4. World Medical Association Declaration of Helsinki. Ethical Principles for Medical Research Involving Human Subjects. 59th WMA General Assembly, Seoul, October 2008.

11 Interpretation and Use of Statistics in Publication

Shreemathi S Mayya

INTRODUCTION

Reporting the results of statistical tests is a topic of concern to researchers of health sciences. They often struggle with choosing the correct statistical procedure and interpreting the results of the statistical test. One way to decide about what should go into the report is to look at published research papers in biomedical journals. They do not contain lots of computer output. They contain the results of the analysis, extracted from the output. It is not necessary to give references for statistics in common use (*t* test , simple chi-square test, Mann-Whitney U-test, etc.) . However, references for the design of the study and higher order statistical methods used in a study should be principally identified with a reference. References for the statistical methods should be to standard works when possible (with pages stated). It is necessary to define statistical terms, abbreviations and symbols, and specify the computer software used (www.icmje.org).

This chapter provides an overview of the correct approach for reporting statistical tests in biomedical journals with examples of correct wording and formatting. All the examples quoted in this chapter are hypothetical. The examples here are worked out in SPSS 10 for Windows (Statistical Package for Social Sciences). Only those outputs required for reporting in a biomedical journal are extracted from the SPSS output. Two tailed test result at 5% level of significance is reported for all the examples. For computation procedure and more details about all these tests, researchers may refer some standard textbooks [Danial(1929); Altman (1990); Bland (2000)].

Depending on the type of data (categorical, quantitative) and shape of the frequency distribution (symmetrical bell shaped, skewed) researchers decide about the descriptive measures, graphs and diagrams, and statistical tests suitable for the presentation and analysis of data.

TESTS FOR CATEGORICAL DATA

Pearson's Chi-square test for nominal data

Requirements

- Qualitative variable with two or more categories
- The data laid out in rows and columns
- The number of observations in each cell of the table must be known
- Frequencies in the different categories should be mutually exclusive and exhaustive.

Situation and Null Hypothesis

Situation1: Independent random samples from two or more populations; Qualitative variable with two or more categories.

Null hypothesis: The distributions of the qualitative variable in different populations are the same or there is no association between row and column variable.

Situation2: Two qualitative variables are being examined in a single sample.

Null hypothesis: Two qualitative variables in a single sample are not associated.

Assumptions

Not more than 20% of the expected values in the cells should be less than 5 and no cell should have an expected value of less than 1.

Example: A college teacher surveyed a simple random sample of 150 male and 200 female undergraduate science students regarding their interest in teaching profession. Here chi-square test was performed to find out whether there is difference in the proportion interested in teaching profession between genders. Results are shown in the table below.

Table 11.1: Interest in teaching profession and gender distribution*

Subject group	Interested in teaching profession		Total
	Interested	*Not interested*	
Male	30 (15)	170 (85)	200(100)
Female	45 (30)	105 (70)	150 (100)

*Number in parenthesis is percentages

Omit column totals, because in this study they do not mean anything. Males and females were sampled as two separate groups. We can quote a test of the null hypothesis that proportion interested in teaching profession is the same in both the gender or there is no association between interest in teaching and gender. This is a large sample and all the expected frequencies are greater than 5 and so, we used the chi-square test, to find out association between gender and interest in teaching.

Reporting: Chi-square test was performed to study the association between gender and interest in teaching profession. The association between these variables was significant, Pearson chi-square= 11.45, df = 1, P= 0.001. Thirty percent of the female students and 15% of the male students expressed interest in teaching (Table 11.1). A difference of 15% (female minus male percent) was observed (95% CI for the difference in percentage: 6.2 to 23.9). Female students were more likely to show interest in teaching profession than male students.

Note: SPSS does not compute confidence interval for the difference in proportion. Here it is calculated with software MedCalc.

Chi-square test of Goodness-of-Fit

A goodness-of-fit test is appropriate when one wishes to decide if an observed distribution of frequencies is incompatible with some preconceived or hypothesized distribution. It requires a sufficient sample size in order for the chi-square approximation to be valid.

Example: Eight hundred and ten toothpaste users were surveyed about their preference to three brands of toothpaste.

Table 11.2: Distribution of preference for three brands of toothpaste

Brand	Number (%)
Brand A	327 (40.4)
Brand B	294 (36.3)
Brand C	189 (23.3)
Total	810 (100)

Reporting: Chi-Square test of goodness-of-fit was performed to determine whether the three brands of toothpaste were equally preferred. Preference for the three brands was not equally distributed in the population, Chi-square=38.457, df=2, P <0.001. Larger percentage of toothpaste users preferred brand A, followed by brand B (Table 11.2).

Chi-square Test for Trend in Proportion

Situation: 2 by K chi-square tables with K ordered categories

If there is a meaningful order to our k groups then the chi-square test for trend provides a more powerful test than the test for nominal categories.

Example: A cross-sectional survey of men aged 40 to 50 years was conducted to collect data on hypertension and BMI. The table below shows the summary.

Table 11.3: Body mass index category and distribution of hypertensive cases*

Hypertensive	Body mass index		
	18.5–25 healthy weight	25–30 overweight	30 or more obese
Yes	20 (4.8)	31 (6.9)	42 (8.4)
No	400 (95.2)	420 (93.1)	460 (91.6)

*Number in parenthesis is percentages

Chi-square test for trend was performed to find out whether there is any linear trend in the proportion of hypertensive cases across the categories of BMI. The test for trend in proportion shows a statistically significant linear trend in the proportion of hypertensive cases across the categories of BMI, Chi-Square test for trend=4.667, df=1, P =0.031. The proportion of hypertensive cases increases with increase in BMI (Table 11.3).

Note: In case of all the abovesaid chi-square tests, whenever the expected frequency is less than 5 in more than 20% of the cells, report *P*-value corresponding to exact test.

McNemar's Test for Paired Data

Situation: 2 × 2 contingency tables with a dichotomous data, two individually matched samples each of sample size n (naturally occurring pairs of observations/two measures taken on the same subject, both on the same scale/two subjects who have been matched or paired on some variable); nominal data.

Assumptions:
• The pairs are mutually independent
• Frequencies in the two categories should be mutually exclusive.

Example: Table 11.4 shows the result of a crossover trial. Researcher wants to know whether drug and placebo are equally effective in relieving headache.

Table 11.4: Intervention and relief of symptoms				
		Time 2 (Placebo)Relief of symptoms (headache) within an hour		
		Yes	No	Totals (Time 1)
Time 1 (Drug)	Yes	a=45(43.3)	b=29(27.9)	a+b=74(71.2)
Relief of symptoms	No	c=8(7.7)	d=22(21.2)	c+d=30(28.8)
(headache) within	Time 2 Totals	a+c=53 (51)	b+d=51(49)	N=104 (100%)
1 hour				

*Number in parenthesis is percentages

The McNemar test examines the difference between the proportions that derived from the marginal sums of the table: P_1(proportion relieved with drug)= (a+b)/N and P_2(proportion relieved with placebo) = (a+c)/N (i.e. P_1= 71.2%, P_2= 51%).

Here we test the null hypothesis that the two proportions in the population, P_1 and P_2 are equal.

Reporting: McNemar's test was performed to determine whether placebo and drug are equally good in relieving headache. Drug was effective in 71.2% of the cases and placebo in 51% of the cases (Table 11.4). The difference in the two proportions were significant; (Exact P = 0.001). Significantly higher percentages of drug treated individuals were relieved of symptoms (drug minus placebo=20.2%, 95% CI: 8.38% to 28.56%)

Note: SPSS does not compute Confidence Interval; here it is calculated with software MedCalc.

TESTS FOR QUANTITATIVE (CONTINUOUS) DATA AND SYMMETRIC DISTRIBUTIONS (PARAMETRIC TESTS)

One-Sample T-Test

Situation: Random sample of size n from a population; quantitative variable.

Assumption: Distribution of the population must be normally or approximately normally distributed.

The null hypothesis tested here is, mean of the population is equal to a given value. It is often a standardized or referenced figure.

Example: The hemoglobin level of a random sample of 10 adult men living in high-altitude were 18, 16, 15, 17,15,18,16,19,16,18 g/dl. Can the researcher conclude from this data that the mean hemoglobin level of adult men living in high-altitude is different from 16 g/dl?

Reporting: One sample t-test was performed to test the null hypothesis that the mean hemoglobin level of adult men living in high-altitude is equal to 16 g/dl. The mean (SD) of hemoglobin level of sample of 10 adult men was 16.8 (1.4) g/dl. The mean hemoglobin level was not significantly different from 16 g/dl (95% CI for mean hemoglobin level 15.8 to 17.8 g/dl, $t_{9\,df}$=1.81, P=0.104). There is no sufficient evidence to conclude on the basis of this data that the mean hemoglobin level of adult men living in high-altitude was different from 16 g/dl.

The two independent sample t-test

Situation: Two independent random samples of size n_1 and n_2 from two populations; quantitative variable.

Assumptions: The populations from which the samples were obtained must be normally or approximately normally distributed. The variances of the populations must be equal.

The null hypothesis tested here is that the means of the two populations are equal, or that the mean difference is zero.

Example: Insulin release in specimens of pancreatic tissue from experimental animals treated with two different stimulants is as follows.

| Stimulant A | 5.70 | 3.67 | 3.98 | 5.65 | 4.48 | 5.82 | 5.96 | 5.43 |
| Stimulant B | 6.89 | 5.33 | 8.28 | 6.12 | 5.65 | 7.76 | 7.12 | |

Here we use independent sample t-test to compare the mean insulin release in animals treated with two different stimulants.

Table 11.5 below shows the summary.

Table 11.5: Insulin release in pancreatic tissue of animals treated with different stimulants

Stimulant	N	Mean	SD
Stimulant A	8	5.086	.903
Stimulant B	7	6.736	1.091

Reporting: Independent sample t-test was applied to test the null hypothesis that mean insulin release in animals treated with two different stimulants is the same.

(Insulin level was recorded to two decimal places, so mean and SD are presented with three decimal places.) The difference in mean insulin level (Stimulant B minus Stimulant A) was 1.649 unit (SE = 0.515, 95% CI 0.538 to 2.761, t_{13df}=3.2, P = 0.007). The study shows good evidence that stimulant B releases more insulin (Table 11.5), and estimate this difference to be between 0.538 and 2.761 units.

The paired t-test

Situation: Two individually matched samples each of sample size n (naturally occurring pairs of observations/two measures taken on the same subject/ two subjects who have been matched or paired on some variable); quantitative variable.

Assumptions: The distribution of the differences between pairs in the population must be independent and normally or approximately normally distributed.

Null hypothesis tested here is that the population means are equal, or that the mean difference is zero.

Example: Following is the pre and postoperative data on creatinine clearance (ml/min) of eight patients anesthetized by halothane:

Subject	1	2	3	4	5	6	7	8
Preoperative	102	88	132	104	112	82	65	92
Postoperative	109	152	135	90	140	118	156	116

Here we use paired sample t-test to compare the mean pre and postoperative creatinine clearance.

Table 11.6 shows the descriptive summary.

Table 11.6: Creatinine clearance (ml/min) of eight patients anesthetized by halothane

	Mean	S. D
Preoperative	97.1	20.3
Postoperative	127.0	22.7

Reporting: Paired sample t-test was performed to test the null hypothesis that mean pre and postoperative creatinine clearance is the same.

The difference in mean creatinine clearance (post minus pre) was 29.9ml/min (SE = 12.1 ml/min, 95% CI 1.4 to 58.4 ml/min, t_{7df} =2.48, P = 0.042). The study shows good evidence that postoperative creatinine clearance was more than preoperative (Table 11.6), and estimates this difference to be between 1.4 and 58.4 ml/min.

One-Way Analysis of Variance (ANOVA)

One-way analysis of variance is an extension of the independent sample t-test to more than two groups. It is a test for the equality of more than two means. Doing t-tests on all possible pairs of k (k>2) means it increases the probability of type I error. An ANOVA controls the overall error by testing all k means against each other at one time.

Assumptions

- The populations from which the samples were obtained must be normally or approximately normally distributed.
- The samples must be independent. (Sample sizes between groups do not have to be equal, but large differences in sample sizes by group may affect the outcome of the multiple comparison tests).
- The variances of the populations must be equal.

Hypotheses

The null hypothesis tested here is that all population means are equal; the alternative hypothesis is that at least one mean is different.

Here we use ANOVA to test the equality of means. A significant ANOVA F-value tells us that the means are not all equal (i.e. reject the null hypothesis). If F-value is significant we have to run a post-hoc comparison test to find out where the differences are—which groups are significantly different from each other and which are not.

Example: Following is the data on unsaturated fatty acids (as a percentage of fats) from three different brands of butter substitutes.

Here we use one way ANOVA to compare the mean fatty acid content of the three brands.

Brand	Fatty Acids (%)						
A	15.2	16.5	14.6	13.7	16.6	15.4	14.5
B	16.8	17.4	16.4	17.2	18.0	17.6	
C	14.6	16.4	14.1	14.2	15.6	14.3	

Interpretation and reporting

Table 11.7 shows the descriptive statistics

Table 11.7: Brand of butter substitutes and Fatty acids (%)

Brand	N	Mean	SD
A	7	15.21	1.06
B	6	17.23	0.57
C	6	14.87	0.93

Reporting

One way ANOVA was performed to test the null hypotheses that mean fatty acids level in all the three brands of butter substitutes are same.

ANOVA test indicated that there was a significant difference in the mean fatty acid level of the three butter substitutes ($F(2, 16) = 12.5$, $P = 0.001$). Descriptive statistics is shown in Table 11.7.

Tukey's procedure was used to conduct pairwise comparisons while controlling the familywise alpha to 0.05. Brand B contains significantly higher level of fatty acid compared to brand A and brand C. Pairwise comparisons among brand A and C were not significant.

The Tukey's procedure was used to calculate simultaneous confidence intervals for the pairwise comparisons while controlling the familywise alpha to 0.05. Table 11.8 shows the descriptive statistics and simultaneous confidence intervals.

Brand	Mean	SD	Comparison	Mean Diff.	P-value	95% CI
A	15.21	1.06	Brand B – Brand A	2.02*	0.002	0.74 to 3.3
B	17.23	0.57	Brand B – Brand C	2.37*	0.001	1.04 to 3.7
C	14.87	0.93	Brand A – Brand C	0.35	0.767	-0.93 to 1.63

Table 11.8: Fatty acids (%) and Tukey's pairwise comparisons

* The mean difference is significant at the 5% level

Note: We proceed to Post-hoc, Tukey's pairwise comparison only when ANOVA F value is significant. Otherwise we report that 'there is no evidence that the brands differ in mean fatty acid level'. If groups have an inherent ordering such as increase in the dose of the drug, then, include an analysis of a trend in the report.

TESTS FOR ORDINAL DATA OR SKEWED DISTRIBUTIONS (NONPARAMETRIC TESTS)

The Mann-Whitney Test

Assumptions
- Two independent random samples of size n_1 and n_2 from their respective populations
- The measurement scale is at least ordinal
- The variable of interest is continuous

Null hypothesis tested here is that the population medians are equal, or that the median difference is zero.

Example: Following is the depression scores recorded for eight patients receiving a new drug and nine patients receiving placebo (with possible values from 0 to 20) in a randomized controlled trial. High scores correspond to states of depression.

Drug	14	11	15	18	12	16	15	17	
Placebo	16	14	19	14	16	17	18	13	16

Here we use Mann-Whitney U test to compare the median depression scores of the two populations.

Table below shows the descriptive summary.

Table 11.9: Treatment and depression scores

	n	Median	IQR	Min.	Max.
Drug	8	15	4.25	11	18
Placebo	9	16	3.5	13	19

Reporting: Mann-Whitney U test was performed to test the null hypothesis that median depression scores of drug and placebo treated groups are the same.

Descriptive summary of depression scores is shown in Table 11.9. The median scores of the two population were not significantly different ($P=0.36$). There is no sufficient evidence to conclude on the basis of this data that the median depression scores in the population of drug and placebo treated groups were different.

Note: Some journals prefer quartiles (Q_1 and Q_3) to IQR in the table

The Wilcoxon matched pairs signed-rank test

Assumptions/requirements

- The sample is random
- The variable is continuous
- The distribution of the differences is symmetric
- The measurement scale is at least interval.

Null hypothesis tested here is that the population medians are equal, or that the median difference is zero.

Example: Following are the scores on attitude towards AIDS patients (with possible values from 0 to 30) before and three months after an intervention programme on attitude to nursing faculties of a hospital.

Before	14	22	20	25	18	16	13	22
After	25	27	21	24	26	24	20	20

Here we perform Wilcoxon's matched pairs signed-rank test to compare the median score before and after intervention.

Table below shows the descriptive summary.

Table 11.10: Attitude scores of eight nurses before and after an intervention program

	Median	IQR	Min.	Max.
Before intervention	19	7.5	13	25
After intervention	24	5.5	20	27

Reporting: Wilcoxon's matched pairs signed-rank test was performed to test the null hypothesis that median attitude scores before and after the intervention programme are same.

Descriptive summary of attitude scores is shown in Table 11.10. The median scores of the two population were not significantly different ($P=0.058$). There is no sufficient evidence to conclude on the basis of this data that the median attitude scores before and after the intervention were different.

Note: Some journals prefer actual quartiles (Q_1 and Q_3) to IQR in the table

For a good discussion of a number of nonparametric tests readers may refer Siegel and Castellan (1988), Conover (1998) and Gibbons (1993).

In scientific research, while reporting statistics, the researcher must include brief as well as adequate information to allow the reader to understand the statistical, result and interpretation. Many aspects are to be taken care of while reporting the results of statistical analysis. Researchers are advised to consult experts for all higher order statistical techniques as they need considerable statistical advice in data collection, analysis, interpretation and reporting. Even for small studies statistical advice before the research begins may be very valuable, especially in helping to match the design to the objectives of the study, and also to give the statistician a greater understanding of the research (Altman, 1981).

Depending on the research questions to be answered and the data available, the researcher decides about the statistical methods to be used for analysis. In the materials and methods section of the scientific paper the researcher has to state the statistical methods used for analysis and the reason why they have been chosen. The findings are to be reported in the results section of research paper and the limitation of analysis if any is to be mentioned in the discussion section. Finally, the conclusions that follow from the findings of the analysis are to be reported in the conclusions section of the paper (Bland, 2005).

GENERAL GUIDELINES FOR REPORTING STATISTICS

- State the level of significance used in statistical tests (alpha) explicitly (commonly set at 0.05)
- 'In medical studies investigators are usually interested in determining the size of difference of a measured outcome between groups, rather than a simple indication of whether or not it is

statistically significant. Confidence intervals present a range of values, on the basis of the sample data, in which the population value for such a difference may lie. P-values - tell you whether there is evidence of a real effect in the population, or not. Confidence intervals - tell you how big the difference might be - regardless of whether the test is statistically significant or not. Preferably both should be presented (Gardner and Altman, 1986)

- Special care should be taken to distinguish between statistical significance and clinical significance. If a study sample is large enough, even small differences can become statistically significant. Confidence intervals may greatly aid interpretation, especially where results are not statistically significant (Altman, 1981)

- Statistics are generally reported to two decimal places, though *P* values are often reported to three places for precision. Exact *P* values, such as *P* = 0.14, are preferable to the term 'N.S.' or 'not significant'. *P* values are preferably quoted to three decimal places, e.g. *P* = 0.021 or *P* = 0.002, but when *P* > 0.1, it is sufficient to keep to two decimal places, e.g. *P* = 0.25. Do not quote P = 0.000 as shown in the SPSS output. Small *P* values can be expressed as *P* < 0.001 or *P* < 0.0001. Both '*p*' and '*P*' are allowed, although the international standard is *P* (large italic). (Fukuda & Ohashi, 1997)

- Whenever a number is less than 0, place a zero before the decimal. For example, use 0.05 instead of .05

- When reporting percentages, include the counts as well. For example, "There were 20% males (10 of 50) represented in the sample." Note also that the percentage was rounded. In general, give percentages as whole numbers if the sample size is less than 100 and to one decimal place if the sample size is larger than 100 (Lang & Secic, 1997, p. 41)

- Whenever multiple comparison statistical tests are performed within the same analysis, adjust alpha level for individual tests to protect overall Type I error rate

- While reporting survey research, include response rate, effects of non-response on the findings and discuss representativeness of the sample.

Reporting the results of statistical tests should be straightforward and simple. Several detailed guidelines on the practice and reporting of statistics in medical papers are available (Altman, Gore, Gardner and Pocock (1983); Altman et al (2001); Bailar and Mosteller (1988); Altman and Bland (1996); Murray(1991)).

SUGGESTED READING

1. Altman DG. Practical Statistics for Medical Research, Chapman and Hall, CRC Press, 1990.
2. Altman DG. Statistics and ethics in medical research. VIII-Improving the quality of statistics in medical journals. Br Med J (Clin Res Ed) 1981; 282(6257): 44-7.
3. Altman DG, Bland JM. Presentation of numerical data. BMJ 1996;312(7030):572.
4. Altman DG, Gore SM, Gardner MJ, Pocock SJ. Statistical guidelines for contributors to medical journals. Br Med J (Clin Res Ed) 1983;286(6376):1489-93.
5. Altman DG, Schulz KF, Moher D, Egger M, Davidoff F, Elbourne D, Gøtzsche PC, Lang T. CONSORT GROUP (Consolidated Standards of Reporting Trials). The revised CONSORT statement for reporting randomized trials: explanation and elaboration Ann Intern Med 2001;134(8):663-94. Review.
6. Bailar JC 3rd, Mosteller F. Guidelines for statistical reporting in articles for medical journals. Amplifications and explanations. Ann Intern Med 1988;108(2):266-73.
7. Bland M. An Introduction to Medical Statistics, 3rd edn. Oxford University Press; 2000.
8. Bland M. Reporting statistical analyses http://www-users.york.ac.uk/~mb55/msc/applbio/statreport/statreport.pdf(accessed on 15/07/2010), 2005.
9. Conover WJ. Practical nonparametric statistics (3rd edn). New York: John Wiley 1998.
10. Daniel, Wayne W. Biostatistics: a foundation for analysis in the health sciences (6th edn) John Wiley & Sons. Inc 1929.
11. Fukuda H, Ohashi Y. A Guideline for Reporting Results of Statistical Analysis in Japanese Journal of Clinical Oncology. Jpn J Clin Oncol 1997;27(3):121-7.
12. Gardner MJ, Altman DG. Confidence intervals rather than P values: estimation rather than hypothesis testing. Br Med J (Clin Res Ed) 1986;292(6522):746-50.
13. Gibbons GD. Nonparametric statistics: An introduction. Newbury Park, CA: Sage 1993.
14. International Committee of Medical Journal Editors [homepage on the Internet]. Uniform Requirements for Manuscripts Submitted to Biomedical Journals: Writing and Editing for Biomedical Publication [accessed on 15/07/2010] Available from: http://www.ICMJE.org.
15. Lang TA, Secic M. How to Report Statistics in Medicine. Philadelphia: American College of Physicians 1997.
16. Murray GD, Statistical guidelines for The British Journal of Surgery. Br J Surg. 1991;78(7):782-4.
17. Siegel S, Castellan NJ. Nonparametric statistics for the behavioural sciences (2nd edn). New York: McGraw-Hill, 1988.
18. Ng KH, Peh WCG. Presenting the statistical results. Singapore Med J 2009; 50:11-14.

12) Preparing Effective Tables

Amar A Sholapurkar

INTRODUCTION

Tables are the most important part of paper. Readers usually judge whether the text is worth reading based on the designing of the tables. Designing will help whether you need more experiments or observations or you need to modify your conclusions. It will help to save your time in writing any unnecessary and extra words. It will also help the reader to grasp the significance of the study quickly without referring the text. You have to remember that tables should convey a clear message. Keep it simpler, short and clear.

Here are two important reasons to think whether one should use tables. First, tables are a means of presenting results in a concise and organized way. They are especially useful if it is difficult to present complicated or too numerous data in the text. Secondly, the cost of publishing tables is too high compared to that of text. Hence, too many tables should not be used.

Three questions come to our mind. "How to", "Whether to" use tables and "What are the general guidelines for preparing tables"? The answer is simple.
1. Tables should be as clear and simple as possible
2. If numerical data is precise then table should be used
3. Tables should be presented when there is large number of data
4. Tables are indicated when large amount of information can be concised and more clearly represented in a tabular rather than in a text form.

DESIGNING THE TABLES

What does a table consist of?

A table consists of a Title, Column headings, Side (row) headings, Body and footnotes. Most of the tables in scientific papers have the pattern as shown in Table 12.1. It is safe to refer the tables [its size, shape, and framework] which are published in the journal you intend to send. Read the instructions to author thoroughly and then design and construct the tables.

Here is the most accepted table format widely accepted in most of the journals (Refer Table 12.1)

- Three horizontal lines are usually used to separate parts of the table. One above the column headings, one below the column headings, and one below the data (To separate the body of the table from the footnotes).
- In tables with subheadings, short horizontal lines are used to group the subheadings under the column heading.
- Avoid the use of additional horizontal and vertical lines [Grid lines] because they give the table a cluttered appearance.
- Remember that most readers read from left to right and hence the results should be presented in columns in which the changes run from the left most columns.

Table 12.1: Title of table

Side heading	Column heading	
	Column subheading (Unit)	Column subheading (Unit)
Row 1	$x_1y_1z_1\ (a_1b_1c_1)$	$X_1Y_1Z_1\ (A_1B_1C_1)$
Row 2	$x_2y_2z_2\ (a_2b_2c_2)$	$X_2Y_2Z_2\ (A_2B_2C_2)$
Row 3	$x_3y_3z_3\ (a_3b_3c_3)$	$X_3Y_3Z_3\ (A_3B_3C_3)$
Row 4	$x_4y_4z_4\ (a_4b_4c_4)$	$X_4Y_4Z_4\ (A_4B_4C_4)$
Row 5	$x_5y_5z_5\ (a_5b_5c_5)$	$X_5Y_5Z_5\ (A_5B_5C_5)$

- Standard errors of the mean are given in parenthesis.
- * Footnote a
- + Footnote b.

Numbering of the Tables

The tables should be numbered in order in which you expect them to appear in the manuscript. Usually arabic numerals (1, 2, 3, 4 ....) is used or sometimes roman numeral (I, II, III, IV ......) which again depends on the guidelines for authors of that particular journal.

Title of the Table

Title is also called as caption or legend. A title should be placed at the top of each table. Make a tentative title where it should convey maximum information as possible about what the table is about. The title should be as short as possible. Let me give some examples of how a table title should be. Please check the tables in the following articles in Australian Dental Journal for the same.

1. P Abbott, SYS Heah. Internal bleaching of teeth: an analysis of 255 teeth. Aust Dent J 2009;54:326-33.
2. AA Sholapurkar, KM Pai, S Rao. Comparison of efficacy of fluconazole mouthrinse and clotrimazole mouth paint in the treatment of oral candidiasis. Aust Dent J 2009;54:341-46.

Remove all redundant words and inconsistent statements. The title should be in such a way that it should be possible to understand the table without referring the text. Here is an example of a concise title.

Incorrect title → Distribution of patients with Diabetes Mellitus, Hypertension, HIV and Acute Leukemia among both the groups.

Correct Title → Distribution of medically compromised patients among both the groups.

How to write Column Headings?

Column headings include (1) headings that identify the items listed in the columns below (2) subheadings (3) units of measurements. It is important to keep the column headings brief.

For experiments that have independent and dependent variables, the independent variables should be in the left column and the dependent variable in the right column. The subheadings are usually to further subdivide column headings into categories [Table 12.1].

Units of Measurements

Units of measurements are usually listed in parenthesis [Table 12.1]. Place them after or below the name of the variable in the column heading/subheading [Table 12.1]. Always use the SI units for measurements. Avoid the use of numerous zeros [For example, use 4 Km rather than 4000 m].

Main Body of the Table

The main body of the table consists of columns (which consists of vertically listed data) and Rows (horizontally listed data). The data should be organized so that the like elements are read down and not across. Here is an example.

Table 12.2: Distribution of medically compromised patients among both the groups

Medically compromised state

		Diabetes Mellitus	HIV	ALL	RT	Steroid therapy	Total
Group A	N = 17	8	0	2	4	3	17
Group B	N = 18	11	2	0	3	2	18

Table 12.3: Distribution of Medically compromised patients among both the groups

Medically compromised state	Group A N = 17	Group B N = 18
Diabetes Mellitus	8	11
HIV	0	2
ALL	2	0
RT	4	3
Steroid therapy	3	2
Total	17	18

Examine Tables 12.2 and 12.3. They are same except that Table 12.2 reads across whereas Table 12.3 reads down. Let me know if you have ever tried to add numbers horizontally rather than vertically? In the same context Table 12.3 is more preferred format as it allows the reader to grasp the information easily. Secondly, it is less space consuming and less expensive to print. Table 12.3 appears smaller than Table 12.2 although the information in both is the same.

Table 12.4: Effects of concentration of intralesional steroids in treatment of oral submucous fibrosis

Concentration	Effect after 8 weeks
1 mg/ml	No
2 mg/ml	No
3 mg/ml	No
4 mg/ml	Yes
5 mg/ml	Yes
6 mg/ml	Yes
7 mg/ml	No
8 mg/ml	No

Table 12.4 is a useless table because it just gives information that the effect of intralesional steroid occurs at concentrations of 4, 5, and 6 mg/ml. Instead it could have been included in the text in a single sentence.

Table 12.5: Comparison of side effects of fluconazole in Group A and B.

	Group		Total
	Group A	Group B	
Total patients	28	29	57
Patient with side effects	2	4	6
Patients without side effects	26	25	51

Table 12.5 is again a useless table and simply space consuming. It can simply be described in the text that 2 patients in Group A and 4 patients in Group B had side effects to the respective drugs.

Note: Indicate statistically significant differences between data by placing symbols. For example, Asterisks (*) after values that are different and then explain the symbols in the footnote.

REQUIREMENTS/INDICATIONS FOR USING A TABLE

- A table should be used when there is lot of data and is difficult to list it in the text
- The table should be small and concise and easily understandable
- Delete unnecessary columns (e.g. Column of P. values) and rows.
- Avoid repetition of information
- Keep brief titles, headings, subheadings and footnote
- Use abbreviations
- Split large tables into two smaller ones
- Use fewer decimal places in measurements and round it up to the nearest decimal. For example, If the measurement is 3.498 cm. then round it up to 3.5 cm instead of using larger decimal places, i.e. give number to the nearest significant figure
- Avoid putting dash [-] in column
- Put zero as '0'
- Insert an * (asterisk) if the term was not measured or if you failed to obtain a value and explain the sign in the footnote
- State which test of significance you used and give p-values, standard deviations or standard errors.

Use of Footnotes

Give appropriate footnotes to your tables. Use the following symbols for footnotes: → *, †, ††, §§, **, etc.

Use of Abbreviations

Always give standard abbreviations. If the abbreviations are not standard then they can be used in the footnotes.

Finally, make sure that the data in the tables agree and matches with the data in the text.

SUGGESTED READING

1. Aydingöz U. Figures, tables, and references: integral but sometimes neglected components of scientific articles. Diagn Interv Radiol 2005;11(2):67-8.

2. Branson RD. Anatomy of a research paper. Respir Care 2004;49(10):1222-8.
3. Brumback RA. Success at publishing in biomedical journals: hints from a journal editor. J Child Neurol 2009;24(3):370-8.
4. Deshpande SB. Art of writing a scientific paper. Indian J Physiol Pharmacol 2006;50(1):1-6.
5. Evans M. Writing a paper. Br J Oral Maxillofac Surg 2007;45(6):485-7.
6. George M Hall. Structure of a scientific paper. In: George M Hall(ed). How to write a Paper. 3rd edn. Noida, India; Byword Viva Publishers Private Limited; 2004. pp. 1-5.
7. Hans-JoaChim Priebe. The results. In: George M Hall (ed). How to write a Paper. 3rd edn. Noida, India; Byword Viva Publishers Private Limited; 2004. 22-35.
8. Kliewer MA. Writing it up: a step-by-step guide to publication for beginning investigators. AJR Am J Roentgenol 2005;185(3):591-6.
9. Kliewer MA. Writing it up: a step-by-step guide to publication for beginning investigators. J Nucl Med Technol 2006;34(1):53-9.
10. Maeve O' Connor, F Peter Woodford. Preparing. In: Maeve O' Connor, F Peter Woodford (eds). Writing Scientific Papers in English. An ELSE-Ciba Foundation Guide for Authors. 1st edn. England : Pitman Medical Publishing Co Ltd; 1977. pp. 7-19.
11. Maeve O' Connor, F Peter Woodford. Writing the first draft. In: Maeve O' Connor, F Peter Woodford (eds). Writing Scientific Papers in English. An ELSE-Ciba Foundation Guide for Authors. 1st edn. England : Pitman Medical Publishing Co Ltd; 1977. pp. 20-28.
12. Michael Derntl. Basics of Research Paper Writing and Publishing, Unpublished manuscript – Revision 2.1 – September 2009.
13. Neill US. How to write a scientific masterpiece. J Clin Invest 2007;117(12):3599-602.
14. Ng KH, Peh WC. Preparing effective tables. Singapore Med J 2009;50(2):117-8; quiz 119.
15. Ng KH, Peh WCG. Writing the results. Singapore Med J 2008;49:856-9.
16. Provenzale JM. Ten principles to improve the likelihood of publication of a scientific manuscript. AJR Am J Roentgenol 2007;188(5):1179-82.
17. Robert A Day. How to Design Effective Tables. In:Robert A Day (ed) How to write and publish a scientific paper. 4th edn. New York: Cambridge University Press; 1995. pp. 59-67.
18. Robert Barrass. Scientists must Write. A guide to better writing for scientists, engineers and students. 1st edn. London: Chapman and Hall, 1978.
19. Setiati S, Harimurti K. Writing for scientific medical manuscript: a guide for preparing manuscript submitted to biomedical journals. Acta Med Indones 2007;39(1):50-5.
20. Sharp D. Kipling's guide to writing a scientific paper. Croat Med J 2002; 43(3):262-7.
21. Temple-Smith M, Goodyear-Smith F, Gunn J. Publish or perish? Evaluation of a writing week. Aust Fam Physician 2009;38(4):257-60.

13 Preparing Effective Illustrations
(Graphs, Photographs, Photomicrographs)

KL Bairy

INTRODUCTION

A good illustration can help the scientist to be heard when speaking or to be read when writing. Illustrations are visual representations of the results obtained from a scientific study. It can help to inform the scientific community the value of the work. It can help to convince the granting agencies to fund the research. There are basically two types of illustrations that are used in scientific papers—graphs and pictorial images such as photographs, images or diagrams. Illustrations are traditionally used to display trends and group results but can also be used to communicate processes or to display detailed data in a simple yet effective manner.

PREPARATION OF GRAPHS

Graphs are a common type of illustration that is often used in scientific papers to present information clearly and effectively, as well as to demonstrate relationship between variable in the data. Before proceeding to the "how to" of graph, let us first examine the question, of "whether to." As a rule, do not construct a graph unless repetitive data must be presented. The reasons are: firstly it is not good science to present a graph of data just because you have them in your workbook; secondly, the cost of publishing graphs can be high compared to that of text and all of us who are involved in publishing scientific literature should worry about cost. Basically the graphs are pictorial tables. There is no need to give both tables as well as graphs in a research article. Certain types of data, particularly sparse type or the type that is monotonously repetitive, do not need to be brought to a graph. Many authors, especially the beginners think that a table, a chart or a graph somehow adds importance to data. They may convert a few data elements in to a graph in order to show that how important the work is. Do not do this. The experienced seniors and journal editors cannot be fooled this way. One has to always remember that any attempt to dress up scientific data may fail miserably. If there is one curve on the proposed graph, one can describe it in words because possibly one value is significant, the rest is window dressing. Rarely there might be a reason to present the same data both in table and a graph, the table presenting the exact values and the graph showing a trend neither otherwise nor apparent. Most editors' will not agree with this, unless the reason for giving both is compelling.

When to use Graph?

Graphs are similar to tables that are used in any scientific communications. The results can be presented as tables or graphs. How to decide which is more effective? This is often a difficult task. A good rule will be this: if the data shows very conclusive trends, making an interesting picture, use a graph. On the other hand if the data are not showing any exciting trend, use a table that is usually easier and cheaper to prepare. Tables are preferred for presenting the exact numbers. In general, it is easy from the graph to grasp the significance or otherwise of data compared to tables.

Organize the graphs in such a manner that they tell a story. Make sure that all graphs are cited in the text. Avoid too many graphs in a paper. Include those graphs that provide essential information that cannot be adequately be described in the text. If graphs are related to one another, then it is common practice to combine them into a composite graph. This saves space and also provides a better picture that allows viewing of the related parts at one site.

How to Prepare Graphs?

This is made easy by the use of computers. Earlier the graphs were prepared by using graph paper, Indian ink, lettering sets etc. making it a cumbersome task. In spite of use of computer software, the principle of producing effective graph is not changed. The size of letter, background, symbols etc. must be such that the published graph is clear and readable. The size of the letter is based on the anticipated reduction that will occur in the publishing process. Use open circle, open triangle, open square, closed circle for reference points (O,Δ, □,●,■). Do not put too many symbols in one graph. If there are many curves in one graph split it in two graphs. Different types of connecting lines (dashed, solid) can be used. The illustrations and legends are separately processed during journal publications. Hence, the legend to the graph or figure should be given on a separate page and not on the top or bottom of the illustrations. One must always refer to Instructions to Authors of a particular journal before preparing a graph as each journal has certain specifications in preparing illustrations. Usually graphs are published in black and white and rarely color graphs are used when it highlights unique information or when it cannot be clearly presented in black and white. It is very expensive to publish graphs in color.

PREPARING EFFECTIVE PHOTOGRAPHS

One has to consider many factors if he/she decides to put a photograph in a research paper. The most important factor is a proper appreciation of the value of the photograph for the article. If photographs are of prime importance one should choose a journal with high quality reproduction standards. In many studies of cell ultra structure, the significance of paper lies in the photograph.

Photographs are used when it is important to show the actual appearance of the object being discussed, such as a biopsy sample, pathology specimen, endoscopic image, patient or patient part. As with the graphs, one must take in to account the column and page width of the journal while deciding the photograph size so that it will fit in journal page. Color photographs are useful for illustrating certain interesting features and are sometimes necessary. Due to high printing costs, color photographs are rarely used. In such cases authors has to bear the cost of production. If subjects or patients photographs are used, the common practice is to hide the identity of the patient by masking the eyes. If disclosure of identity is unavoidable, then written, informed consent should be obtained from the subject/patient prior to taking photograph and a copy of the consent letter should be sent to the journal along with manuscript submission.

Submission Format

Generally journal editors will ask the authors to submit the photographs as glossy prints. Of late the journals ask to submit the photograph electronically. For more details you are advised to look in to instructions to authors of their target journals. File should be saved in either TIFF or EPS formats. Other image file formats, e.g. JPG, GIF, BMP, and Microsoft powerpoint slides. If the files cannot be saved in TIFF or EPS, it may be saved in JPG at the highest resolution.

Cropping

Sometimes the quality of the photograph is not that good but you want it to be published legibly. This is possible if you take some special care. Instead of including the whole photo, crop the photograph to include only important part. If the photograph is in digital format you can crop it electronically. If you are submitting a print, you can write, "crop marks" on the margin to show where the photograph should be cropped. Significant reduction in photographs size should be avoided and greatest fidelity of reproduction results when one furnishes exact photographs, requiring neither reduction nor enlargement.

Necessary Keys and Guides

Superimposing arrows or letter can draw the reader's attention to the significant features, making it easy to construct meaningful legends. This is often done if one cannot crop down to the features of special interest. Figure 13.1 shows arrow marks used to highlight different sizes of NORS.

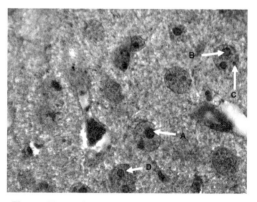

Figure 13.1: NORs in Liver (100 x)
A – Regular shaped NOR
B – Large sized NOR
C – Small sized NOR
D – Medium sized NOR

Most of the journal request for electronic submission. If you are submitting a print, mark "top" on what you considered to be the top of the photograph. Mark it on the back with a soft pencil and also write the name of the first author so that in case the photograph is misplaced by the publishers or editors this will help them to trace it. You can also indicate the preferred location for each photograph so that one can be sure all illustrations are referred to in the text in order.

Legend to Illustrations

A clear, descriptive legend must be provided for each illustration (whether it is table, photograph, radiological image or diagram). Each legend should explain concisely as much information as possible about what the illustration tells the readers. It should be able to standalone so that the reader need not refer the text to understand the illustrations.

SUMMARY

Illustrations such as tables, photographs, radiological images or diagrams are important and useful tools for better understanding a scientific paper as they make visual impact. Authors should follow the guidelines issued by specific journal while preparing illustrations for publications.

SUGGESTED READING

1. Aydingöz U. Figures, tables, and references: integral but sometimes neglected components of scientific articles. Diagn Interv Radiol 2005;11(2):67-8.
2. Ng KH, Peh WCG. Preparing effective illustrations. Part 1: graphs. Singapore Med J 2009;50:245-9.
3. Ng KH, Peh WCG. Preparing effective illustrations. Part 2: photographs, images and diagrams. Singapore Med J 2009;50:330-35.

Writing the Results

Wilfred CG Peh and Kwan-Hoong Ng

INTRODUCTION

The Results section of a scientific paper is the third component of the conventional IMRAD (Introduction, Materials and methods, Results and Discussion) structure of an original article. This section aims to provide answers to the research question, i.e. "What was found?"

The Results section can be divided into two components, namely: Presentation of main data collected from the research done and observations made and interpretation of analyzed data.

Information contained in this section should not overlap with contents of the Introduction, Materials and Methods and Discussion sections. As with other aspects of manuscript preparation, authors should always check the individual journal's "Instructions to Authors" or "Author Guidelines" for details of in-house style requirements.

PRESENTING THE RESULTS

The steps to presenting the results can be divided into three phases, namely: collect, analyze and interpret. Begin by reviewing all the collected data, and determine which data to present. The results that are relevant to the research question, i.e. purpose of the study, should be identified. The outcomes for every item mentioned in the materials and methods section should be given, i.e. there should be a direct match. A good practice is to start working on the results section as soon as the data collection is completed. Analysis includes data summaries (including descriptive statistics) and application of statistical tests to data.

Raw data (such as patient records, individual observations and various measurements) should not be included in the manuscript. If this is considered to be very important, then consider adding an appendix to list these items. Ensure that the data is accurate and consistent. If the data differences are statistically significant, actual figures should be provided. When reporting results of statistical tests, any assumption that has been made should be explicated stated. The effects of variables using measures that are clinically relevant should be reported. The appropriate number of significant figures to report the means and other measured or calculated values should be used. The significant figures should accurately reflect the degree of precision of the original measurement. Exact p-values should be reported (Example 1). Reviewers and readers should be able to independently evaluate, analyze and verify the data presented. Finally, enlisting the help of a biostatistician to review the statistical analysis, and the presentation and interpretation of the results, is recommended.

USE OF TABLES AND ILLUSTRATIONS TO PRESENT RESULTS

The results should be presented, by default, in text format. Depending on the nature of data, consider using tables, and illustrations such as graphs, diagrams and images, as some data are better presented using these means. Tables are used to present information in a concise, detailed and precise manner. They help make a manuscript more readable by summarizing both numerical data and statistical results from research done (Example 2). Presenting data in a table rather than part of the text is also an effective way to reduce the length of the manuscript. Data suitable for presentation in table format include: precise numerical data rather than proportions or trends, large numbers of related data, clearer summary of information in tabular form rather than descriptive text, and complex information. Tables should be self-explanatory and do not duplicate data given in the text or graphs.

Illustrations (or figures) are visual representations of results obtained, and can be divided into graphs (Example 3) and pictorial images such as diagrams, radiological images and photographs. Illustrations functions to communicate study findings by providing visual impact. Graphs aim to present data that is too complicated to be described in the text and demonstrate relationships between variables in the data. Graphs are also able to reveal patterns or trends in the data. Depending on the kind of data to be presented, the appropriate type of graph should be selected, including: scattergrams (for independent and dependent numeric variables), bar charts (for dependent numeric variables), and bar charts or pie charts (for proportions).

Illustrations provide visual information and may effectively improve the readability of a manuscript. Common types of illustrations include: patient or specimen photographs (e.g. clinical, intraoperative, endoscopic, laparoscopic, intraoral and enteroscopic photographs), photomicrographs (including optical and electron micrographs) (Example 4), radiological images (e.g. radiograph, computed tomography, magnetic resonance imaging, ultrasonography, angiography and radionuclide imaging) (Example 4), physiological signal tracings (e.g. electrocardiography, electroencephalography, echocardiography), laboratory graphs (e.g. chromatogram and karyogram), and line drawings (e.g. flow chart, algorithm, schematic diagram and chemical structure) (Example 5). Illustrations should be submitted in a format that will allow high-quality reproduction. It is important to maintain patient confidentiality, particularly for photographs. The identity of patients should be hidden. If disclosure of identity is unavoidable, then written informed consent should be obtained from the patient or guardian prior to manuscript submission.

ORGANIZING THE RESULTS

When embarking on writing the Results section, one should first decide on the sequence. Many authors start with reprising the research question. The most important results should be listed first. If tables or illustrations have been created, key points from each table or graph can be used as a basis for writing the Results section. Tables and other illustrations should be numbered consecutively in the same chronological sequence of appearance in the text. Conventionally, past tense is used for this section. The tables and illustrations should stand-alone, with legends (or captions) that provide a clear description and contain all pertinent information. By convention, legends appear above tables and below figures and graphs.

COMMON PROBLEMS

- Illogical sequence of presentation
- Inaccurate data
- Data repetition: among text, table, graphs and other illustrations
- Expected data not reported
- Misplaced information
- Too much data/ raw data
- Use of statistical significance to prove clinical significance
- Making the assumption that a non-significant result proves the null hypothesis

- Overuse and abuse of illustrations
- Attempts to discuss and draw conclusions
- Tables listed are not cited in the text
- Data in tables do not agree with data given in the text
- Wrong type of graph is chosen to represent the data
- Graph is not plotted to scale
- Misuse of pseudo three-dimensional graphs

SUMMARY

The Results section should present relevant collected data arising from the Materials and Methods section and provide the authors' interpretation of the analyzed data. This section consists primarily of text, and if necessary, may be complemented by tables, figures and other illustrations. Tables are used to make a scientific manuscript more readable by summarizing numeric data from the text, and aid in presenting complex data in a concise and organized manner. Illustrations such as graphs and images help improve the readability by presenting data with a visual impact. The flow of tables and illustrations, in relation to text, should be able to tell a logical story.

EXAMPLES

Example 1: Actual p-values are given in this table*

Table 14.1: Univariate analysis of variables affecting the outcome

Variable	p-value	
	Lysholm	IKDC
Age at surgery	0.59	0.32
Presence of associated meniscal injury	0.43	0.48
Tibial tunnel position in the coronal plane	0.31	0.12
Tibial tunnel position in the sagittal plane	<0.01	<0.01
Femoral tunnel position in the coronal plane	0.19	0.25
Femoral tunnel position in the sagittal plane	0.39	0.28
Coronal angle of tibial tunnel	0.32	0.27

IKDC: International Knee Documentation Committee

Example 2: Use of table to summarize numerical data and statistical results**

---

* *Reproduced with permission from: Avadhani A, Rao PS, Rao SK. Effect of tibial tunnel position on arthroscopically-assisted anterior cruciate ligament reconstruction using bone-patellar tendon-bone grafts: a prospective study. Singapore Med J 2010;51(5):413-7.*

** *Reproduced with permission from: Shakiba M, Sadr S, Nefei Z, et al. Combination of bolus dose vitamin D with routine vaccination in infants: a randomized trial. Singapore Med J 2010;51(2):440-5.*

Table 14.2: Distribution of 25-OH vitamin D levels in the three groups of infants who received different doses of vitamin D

	Amount of vitamin D supplement		
	200 IU daily (I)	400 IU daily (II)	50,000 IU bolus/ 2 mths (III)
No. of infants	19	26	30
Mean 25-OH serum level + SD	31.3 ± 8.5	38.4 ± 11.4	53.7 ± 19.5
(range) (ng/ml)	(20-51)	(23-64)	(28-102)

One-way ANOVA: p = 0.001: Tukey's test: (I) vs. (II): vs (III) p = 0.5 (I) vs (III): p= 0.001; (II) vs (III) p = 0.005)
25.OH: 25 hydroxy. S.D. standard deviation

Example 3: Use of bar chart*

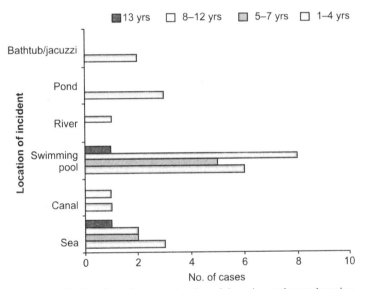

Figure 14.1: Bar chart shows the location of drowning and near-drowning cases based on age

Example 4: Mammograms and photomicrographs used as illustrations**

---

* *Reproduced with permission from: Tyebally A, Ang SY. Kids can't float: epidemiology of paediatric drowning and near-drowning in Singapore. Singapore Med J 2010; 51(5): 429-33.*

** *Reproduced with permission from: Muttarak M, Kongmebhol P, Sukhamwang N. Breasts calcifications: which are malignant? Singapore Med J 2010; 50(9):907-14.*

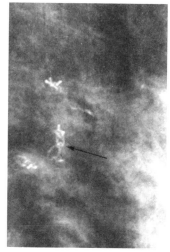

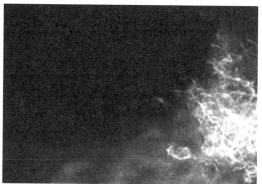

Figure 14.2: Left mediolateral oblique mammogram shows the knots in the calcified suture material (arrow)

Figure 14.3: Magnified view of left mediolateral oblique mammogram

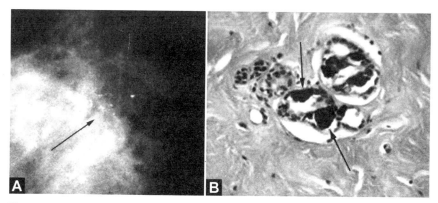

Figures 14.4A and B: A. Magnification view shows a group of amorphous calcifications (arrow). B. Photomicrograph shows fibrocystic change with calcifications in the lumen (arrows) (Hematoxylin and eosin, × 40)

Example 5: Flow diagram used as an illustration*

* *Reproduced with permission from: Lee WS, Chai PF, Boey CM, Looi LM. Aetiology and outcome of neonatal cholestasis in Malaysia. Singapore Med J 2010;50(5):434-9.*

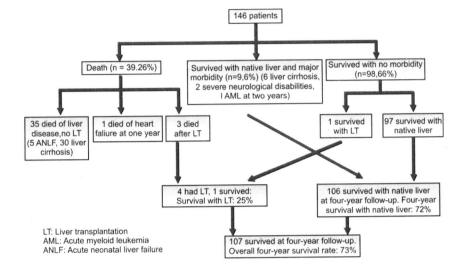

Figure 14.5: Outcomes of 146 patients with neonatal cholestasis

SUGGESTED READING

1. Ng KH, Peh WCG. Preparing effective illustrations. Part 1: graphs. Singapore Med J 2009;50:245-9.
2. Ng KH, Peh WCG. Preparing effective illustrations. Part 2: photographs, images and diagrams. Singapore Med J 2009;50:330-5.
3. Ng KH, Peh WCG. Preparing effective tables. Singapore Med J 2009; 50:117-9.
4. Ng KH, Peh WCG. Presenting the statistical results. Singapore Med J 2009; 50:11-4.
5. Ng KH, Peh WCG. Writing the results. Singapore Med J 2008;49:856-9.
6. Peh WCG, Ng KH. Basic structure and types of scientific papers. Singapore Med J 2008;49:522-5.

15 How to Write the Discussion and Conclusion

Wilfred CG Peh and Kwan-Hoong Ng

INTRODUCTION

The discussion section is the last component of the conventional IMRAD (Introduction, materials and methods, results and discussion) structure of an original article. This section aims to provide answers to "what do the findings mean?" by answering the research question posed at the end of the Introduction section, stating the major findings of the study, and explaining how the results support the answers and fit in with existing knowledge. Many authors find this section the most difficult to write, probably as this section requires the most "originality" and organization, such that the thoughts of the authors' are conveyed in a logical and easily-comprehensible flow. To achieve this, several rewritten drafts are often required.

It is important to keep focused and to bear in mind that this section aims to discuss and not repeat the major findings of the study. Authors should avoid the temptation to pack in too much information, particularly extraneous information that may not be directly relevant to the objectives of the study. The discussion section should encompass the following items: emphasize new and important aspects of the study, its relation to previous work done, implications of the current work, weaknesses or limitations of the current study, suggestions for future research, and the conclusion.

COMPONENTS OF THE DISCUSSION

New and important aspects of the study should be emphasized, but avoid repeating detailed data or other material from the Introduction, Materials and Methods, and Results sections. Condensing the main findings of the study into one to two sentences that form the opening statements of the discussion section is encouraged (Example 1). When discussing each new finding, provide evidence for each individual finding.

It is expected that a thorough literature search has been performed, in order to adequately provide relationship of findings from the current study to what has been previously reported by others. There is, however, no need to quote every single reference that has been found. Only sound and relevant work should be quoted, omitting those studies of low clinical impact and lacking scientific rigor. Contradictory and unexpected findings from the authors' study should be identified and highlighted, and then discussed and explained, particularly discrepancies (Example 2). The creed "honesty is the best policy" holds true when attempting to explain data that does not quite fit.

An attempt should be made to highlight the implications of the current work, particularly if there is any clinical and scientific impact. If there are new findings, the authors should try to explore possible mechanisms or explanations, and state new hypotheses, if any. Potential alteration of existing practice or contributions to progress and understanding in the field of study should be listed and discussed. The authors should provide their own insights, suggest further areas of study, state any plans to expand on their work and areas of future research (Example 3). For recommendations for future areas of research, specifics (rather than general statements) should be provided with a stated purpose.

It is expected that authors objectively mention the weaknesses and limitations of the current study (Example 4). These include small sample size, retrospective nature of the study, and problems with the methods or investigative tools. If unusual methods were used, explanations should be provided. How these methodology pitfalls influenced the validity of the results or their interpretation should be discussed.

The conclusion should be succinct and be a precise summary of the most important findings, and is linked with the goals of the study. Ideally, a clear take-home message should be provided (Example 5). The conclusion is often the last paragraph of the Discussion section, although in some journals, the Conclusion may be a separate section.

COMMON PROBLEMS

- Overlong or irrelevant discussion
- Repetition of data from the Results section
- Introduction of new data in this section
- Failure to discuss importance of findings
- Misinterpretation of results (leading to faulty conclusions)
- Unqualified statements
- Conclusion is not supported by data

- Failure to identify any weaknesses of the study
- Excessive quoting and discussion of irrelevant references
- Preferential quoting of references
- Omission of key references
- Claiming unwarranted priority
- Alluding to work that has not been completed
- Making statements on economic benefit and cost, without obtaining appropriate economic methodology, data and analysis.

SUMMARY

The Discussion section aims to answer the research question, emphasize new and important aspects of the study, provide the authors' interpretation of the meaning of the study findings, highlight study weaknesses, and suggest areas of future research. There should be a succinct conclusion supported by original data, with a clear take-home message.

EXAMPLES

Example 1: The opening statement of Discussion states the main study finding, followed by comparison with previously-published work*

Overall, the level of mental health knowledge of the general public is considerably low. The current finding is not dissimilar to previous studies done on knowledge of mental health using different tools and different population groups which concluded that lay people generally have a poor understanding of mental illness; they were unable to correctly recognize and identify the mental problems, did not understand the underlying causal factors, were fearful of those perceived as mentally ill, had incorrect beliefs about the effectiveness of treatment interventions, and were often reluctant to seek help from mental health professionals.

Example 2: Explanation of contradictory findings**

In the present study, a low-risk of GCA was observed in patients who have a high intake of pulses. This could be the reason for the low

---

Reproduced with permission from: Yeap R, Low WY. Mental health knowledge, attitute and help-seeking tendency: a Malaysian context. Singapore Med J 2009;50(12):1169-76.

**Reproduced with permission from: Sumathi B, Ramalingam S, Navaneethan U, Jayanthi V. Risk factors for gastric cancer in South India. Singapore Med J 2009;50(2):147-51.*

incidence of GCA in North India, where pulses are consumed in large amounts compared to South India, where the consumption of pulses is much lower. The staple food for the people of South India is rice and it has been shown to be an independent risk factor for GCA in another case-control study from the southern part of India. However, we did not identify rice as a risk factor for GCA. Smoking as a variable risk factor for GCA has been reported from India. However, smoking did not predict the development of GCA in the present study. The results were contradictory in another study from the same city, which however consisted of a heterogeneous population. This could probably be attributed to cigar smoking rather than cigarette smoking being more common in this part of the country, and explain the noncontribution of smoking as a major risk factor. In addition, there was no significant association between betel quid chewers and GCA.

Example 3: Authors' explanations for their findings and suggestions for further areas of study*

The present study thus demonstrated the chemopreventive efficacy of curcumin and piperine in DMBA-induced hamster buccal pouch carcinogenesis. The chemopreventive potential of curcumin and piperine are probably due to their antilipid peroxidative and antioxidant potential or modulating effect on the carcinogen detoxification process. Further studies are, however, required in order to better understand the underlying mechanisms of the chemopreventive actions of curcumin and piperine.

Example 4: Stating study limitations**

There were several limitations in the present study. This series of patients was enrolled from a single institution, and the data was retrospectively reviewed. The small number of patients may also mask several other important factors that could be accountable for the outcomes identified. Although these limitations are significant, this study remains important in reviewing the numerous issues surrounding the management of diaphragmatic rupture after blunt trauma.

---

* *Reproduced with permission from: Manoharan S, Balakrishnan S, Menon VP, et al. Chemopreventive efficacy of curcumin and piperine during 7,12-dimethylbenz[a] anthracene-induced hamster buccal pouch carcinogenesis. Singapore Med J 2009;50(2):139-46.*
** *Reproduced with permission from: Tan KK, Yan ZY, Vijayan A, Chiu MT. Management of diaphragmatic rupture from blunt trauma. Singapore Med J 2009;50(12):1150-3.*

Example 5: Conclusion and take-home message*

In conclusion, selenium intake and status are related to breast cancer risk. Therefore, selenium intake through the diet should be emphasized as a chemopreventive agent in reducing the risk of breast cancer. There is an urgent need to analyze the selenium content in Malaysian foods.

SUGGESTED READING

1. Hess DR. How to write an effective discussion. Respir Care 2004;49(10):1238-41.
2. International Committee of Medical Journal Editors. Uniform requirements for manuscripts submitted to biomedical journals: writing and editing for biomedical publications. Updated October 2008. Available at: www.icmje.org
3. Kliewer MA. Writing it up: a step-by-step guide to publication for beginning investigators. AJR Am J Roentgenol 2005;185(3):591-6.
4. Naik SR, Aggarwal R. 'Introduction' and 'discussion' in a scientific paper. J Assoc Physicians India 1991;39(9):703-4.
5. Ng KH, Peh WCG. Writing the discussion. Singapore Med J 2009;50:458-61.
6. Peh WCG, Ng KH. Basic structure and types of scientific papers. Singapore Med J 2008;49:522-5.
7. Szklo M. Quality of scientific articles. Rev Saude Publica 2006;40 Spec no: 30-5.

---

* Reproduced with permission from: Suzana S, Cham BG, Ahmad Rohi G, et al. Relationship between selenium and breast cancer: a case-control study in the Klang Valley. Singapore Med J 2009;50(3):265-9.

16 Quoting the References

Keerthilatha M Pai
Amar A Sholapurkar

INTRODUCTION

Honest and professional citation of references provides part of the framework for sound written research. Whenever you draw upon previously published work, you must acknowledge the source. Any information not from your experiment and not "common knowledge" should be recognized by a citation. How citations are presented varies considerably from discipline to discipline and you should refer to 'instructions to authors' for the specific journal. Quotes that appear in the article, if long, should have their own indented paragraph, otherwise if they are in the natural flow of the article should be within speech marks, and in both cases they should include a reference. Avoid references that are difficult to find, and/or refer to papers not written in the language of the journal to which you are submitting your paper.

The References section that appears at the end of the paper includes all references cited in your paper. This is in contrast to a bibliography, common in books, where works read but not necessarily cited in the text are listed. The order in which references are presented also varies from journal to journal and you should consult the journal's 'instructions to authors'.

DEFINITION OF A BIBLIOGRAPHICAL REFERENCE

A set of data or elements describing a document or part of a document and sufficiently precise and detailed to enable a potential reader to identify and locate it.

A typical reference citation should:
- Identify the source precisely
- Describe it sufficiently
- Guide the readers adequately if they wish to obtain the document.

WHY CITE REFERENCES?

- To acknowledge the sources you have used to establish your arguments and criticisms
- To enable others to identify and trace the sources you have used for your ideas
- To avoid plagiarism.

WHAT IS ITS PURPOSE?

The purpose is to describe your sources in an accurate and consistent manner and to indicate within the text of your paper where the particular sources were used.

REFERENCES: MUCH ADO ABOUT NOTHING

- Examiners infer that sloppy references may indicate sloppy work
- Check, re-check and re-re-check
- It is easy to check and find mistakes.

WHAT KIND OF INFORMATION NEEDS A REFERENCE?

Do not give references for facts which are well known:
a. Dental caries is a microbial disease (no reference needed)
b. The accuracy of CBCT images is high in linear measurements (give reference).

COMPONENTS TO CITING REFERENCES

There are two components to citing references:
- The way you acknowledge, cite the source in your text
- The way you list your sources at the end of your work to enable identification, i.e. bibliography/reference list.

WHICH SOURCES CAN BE USED FOR REFERENCING?

- Use textbooks, review articles, original papers from journals, electronic sources—any source which can be authenticated
- Preferably, do not use newspaper clippings, articles "in press"; personal communication.

SOME TIPS FOR REFERENCING

- Never cite a reference which you have not read
- Be consistent and accurate

- Do not cite from abstracts—read the full article
- File all references—hard copy/electronic.

TWO MAJOR SYSTEMS OF CITING REFERENCES

1. Vancouver system
2. Harvard system

VANCOUVER SYSTEM*

Vancouver, a "numbered" style, follows rules established by the International Committee of Medical Journal Editors <http://www.icmje.org/>. It is also known as: Uniform Requirements for Manuscripts Submitted to Biomedical Journals.

- Most common system at present
- References are numbered consecutively in the order in which they are first mentioned in the text
- Identify references in text, tables, and legends by Arabic numerals in parentheses
- The titles of journals should be abbreviated according to the style used in Index Medicus
- Less obtrusive
- Saves the reader time used in searching.

Journal Article

For journal articles the required elements for a references are:

Author's surname first, followed by the initial(s). Title of article. Title of Journal [abbreviated]. Year of publication month date;Volume number(Issue number):Page numbers. Refer Box 16.1 for details.

Source—*Monash University library, "Vancouver style (uniform requirements for manuscripts submitted to biomedical journals)" libweb@lib.monash.edu.au, Available at http://www.lib.monash.edu.au/tutorials/citing/vancouver.html, Accessed: 30 July 2010.*

Dave O Malley, Guide to the Vancouver system of referencing, Available at http://www.fgdp.org.uk/pdf/vancouver.pdf, Accessed: 30 July 2010.

Box 16.1

- The name of the author should be given with the surname first, followed by the initial(s). There should be no punctuation or space between the initials.
- Where there is more than one author, the names should be separated by a comma and a space. The last author's initial(s) should be followed by a full stop.
- Where the work is anonymous, no author should be cited. "Anon" and similar are not used in the Vancouver system.
- Where there are more than six authors, only the first six should be listed, followed by "et al".
- Where the work is credited to an organization, the name of the organization should be given in full, as it was at the time of authorship.
- Abbreviate the title according to the style used in Medline. Lists of abbreviations can be found via http://www.ncbi.nlm.nih.gov/entrez/citmatch_help.html#JournalLists. Use no punctuation (other than spaces) in the abbreviated journal name.
- The year should be followed by the publication month and/or date, where available or necessary. This will depend on the frequency of the journal.
- The issue number may be omitted if the page numbering is continuous throughout issues in a given volume.

Examples

- Halpern SD, Ubel PA, Caplan AL. Solid-organ transplantation in HIV-infected patients. N Engl J Med 2002;347(4):284-7.
- Bergdahl J, Anneroth G, Perris H. Cognitive therapy in the treatment of patients with resistant burning mouth syndrome: a controlled study. J Oral Pathol Med 1995;24(5):213-5.

Books

The required elements for a book reference are:

Author/Editor/Compiler's surname Initials. Title of the book. # ed.[if not 1st] Place of publication: Publisher's name; Year of publication. Refer **Box 16.2** for details.

Box 16.2

- Where the named author is the editor of the book, the author's name should be followed by a comma and "editor(s)" as applicable and then followed by full stop. Do not abbreviate this to "ed" as this denotes edition number.
- Only first words of the article title and words that normally begin with a capital letter are capitalized. Title is followed by full stop.
- For books which have an edition number, the title should be followed by a full stop, followed by the edition number in numerals, followed by " ed" and then a full stop.
- The place of publication should be a town or city followed by colon
- Write the Publisher/ Company name followed by semicolon.
- Finally write the year of publication followed by a full stop
- In case of Book chapter where page numbers are given, insert a space after the full stop after the date, followed by "p." and the page numbers.

Examples

- Robert A Day, (editor). How to write and publish a scientific paper. 4th edn. New York: Cambridge University Press 1995.

- Murray PR, Rosenthal KS, Kobayashi GS, Pfaller MA (editors). Medical microbiology. 4th edn. St Louis: Mosby 2002.

Book Chapters

The required elements for a book reference are:

Author's surname initials. Title of chapter. In: Editor's surname Initials, editor. Title of the book. # ed.[if not 1st] Place of publication: Publisher's name; Year of publication. p. #. [page numbers of chapter]
- Abbreviate page numbers to p., e.g. p. 126-35.
- Abbreviate numbers where appropriate e.g. p. 152-8.

Example: Meltzer PS, Kallioniemi A, Trent JM. Chromosome alterations in human solid tumors. In: Vogelstein B, Kinzler KW (editors). The genetic basis of human cancer. New York: McGraw-Hill; 2002. pp 93-113.

Journal Article on the Internet

The required elements for a reference are:

Author's surname, Author's name initials. Title of article. Abbreviated Title of Journal [serial on the Internet]. Year of publication Month day [cited Year Month Day];Volume Number(Issue number):[about number of pages or screens]. Available from: URL
- Only cite month/day if applicable
- Can list either pages or screens

Example: Abood S. Quality improvement initiative in nursing homes: the ANA acts in an advisory role. Am J Nurs [serial on the Internet]. 2002 Jun [cited 2002 Aug 12];102(6):[about 3 p.]. Available from: http://www.nursingworld.org/AJN/2002/ june/Wawatch.htm

Web Pages

The format for citing web pages is as follows (non-bold fields may not apply):

[Author]. [Title of document.] **[Title of web site]. Available at: [URL]. Accessed: [Date].**

Example: National Institute for Health and Clinical Excellence. Donepezil, galantamine, rivastigmine (review) and memantine for the treatment of Alzheimer's disease (amended). National Institute for Health and Clinical Excellence site. Available at: http://guidance.nice.org.uk/TA111/guidance/pdf/English/download.dspx. Accessed: Oct 1, 2007

Harvard System*

- This system uses the primary author's last name and year of publication in the body of the text
- The reference list is arranged alphabetically by the author's names.

Journal Articles

For journal articles the required elements for references are:
  Author, Initials., Year. Title of article. *Full Title of Journal*, Volume number (Issue/Part number), Page numbers.

Example — Annas, G.J., 1997.New drugs for acute respiratory distress syndrome.*New England Journal of Medicine*, 337(6), pp. 435-439.

Journal Articles from an Electronic Source

The required elements for a reference are:
  Author, Initials., Year. Title of article. *Full Title of Journal*, [type of medium] Volume number (Issue/Part number), Page numbers if available.

  Available at: include web site address/URL(Uniform Resource Locator) and additional details of access, such as the routing from the home page of the source. [Accessed date].

Example: Boughton, J.M., 2002. The Bretton Woods proposal: an in depth look. *Political Science Quarterly*, [Online]. 42 (6),

Available at: Blackwell Science Synergy http://www.pol.upenn/articles [Accessed 12 June 2005].

Book Reference

The required elements for a book reference are:
  Author, Initials/First name., Year. *Title of book*. Edition. Place of publication: Publisher.

Example: Conover, W. J., 1998. *Practical nonparametric statistics*. 3rd edn. New York: John Wiley.

---

* Source — *Anglia Ruskin University, "Guide to the Harvard Style of Referencing", Harvard System of Referencing Guide site, Available at http://libweb.anglia.ac.uk/referencing/harvard.htm. Accessed: 30 July 2010.*

WHICH SYSTEM SHOULD I CHOOSE?

Vancouver Format

Uniform Requirements for Manuscripts Submitted to Biomedical Journals: Writing and Editing for Biomedical Publication.

Journals which follow the ICMJE guidelines will accept papers if the references are in theVancouver format.

International Committee of Medical Journal editors (ICMJE) www.icmje.org

References in the Introduction

- Support statement of the problem
- Previous work done in that topic
- Chronological order
- No need to start with references to mythology
- If citing from another reference (and not from the original source), say so.

References in the Materials and Methods Section

- If a method/technique is very well established and known—no need to give a reference
- Variations in established method/technique require references
- Uncommon statistical methods—require references

References in the Discussion Section

- References of comparative studies
- If your results differ from others' work due to differences in techniques–give references for those methods/techniques
- References should be current (include all *pertinent latest* references)
- Remember to search nonindexed journals too!

Abbreviations

These are commonly used abbreviations:
- **c.** = circa (about, approximately)
- **ch.** = chapter
- **edn.** = edition
- **et al.** = and others
- **fig; figs** = figure(s)
- **ill ills** = illustrator(s)

- **p.** = page(s)
- **para paras** = paragraph(s)
- **pt pts** = part(s)
- **rev** = revised
- **suppl** = supplement
  Check journal abbreviations in: *PubMed Journals Database*

SUGGESTED READING

1. Uniform requirements for manuscripts submitted to biomedical journals: writing and editing for biomedical publication [homepage on the Internet]. Philadelphia, PA:International Committee of Medical Journal Editors; [updated 2003 Nov; cited 2004 Oct 9]. Available from: http://www.icmje.org.
2. Style manual for authors, editors and printers. 6th ed. Milton, Qld: John Wiley & Sons; 2002. Monash holdings.
3. Patrias K. National Library of Medicine recommended formats for bibliographic citation. SUPPLEMENT: Internet Formats [monograph on the Internet]. Bethesda, MD: U.S. Dept. of Health and Human Services, Public Health Service, National Institutes of Health; 2001 [cited 2007 May 23]. 106 p. Available from: http://www.nlm.nih.gov/pubs/formats/internet2001.pdf.
4. Monash University library, "Vancouver style (uniform requirements for manuscripts submitted to biomedical journals)" libweb@lib.monash.edu.au, Available at http://www.lib.monash.edu.au/tutorials/citing/vancouver.html, Accessed: 30 July 2010.
5. Dave O Malley, Guide to the Vancouver system of referencing, Available at http://www.fgdp.org.uk/pdf/vancouver.pdf, Accessed: 30 July 2010.
6. Anglia Ruskin University, "Guide to the Harvard Style of Referencing", Harvard System of Referencing Guide site, Available at http://libweb.anglia.ac.uk/referencing/harvard.htm. Accessed: 30 July 2010.

17 Writing the Acknowledgments

Nirmala N Rao

INTRODUCTION

Acknowledgments embody a wide range of relationships among people, agencies institutions and research. Moreover, acknowledgments are arguably more personal, singular, or private expressions of appreciation and contribution. Just as citation indexing proved to be an important tool for evaluating research contribution, acknowledgment can be considered as metric parallel to citations in the academic audit process.

CATEGORIES OF ACKNOWLEDGMENT

Acknowledgment in scientific articles may be made for a number of reasons but often implies a significant intellectual debt. Cronin et al have proposed six categories of acknowledgment and they are:

1. Moral support
2. Financial support
3. Editorial support
4. Presentational support
5. Instrumental/technical support
6. Conceptual support or peer interactive communication (PIC)

Of all the categories, PIC has been considered to be the most important for identifying intellectual obligation. While some researchers have considered acknowledgement of PIC is as valuable as citation. However, acknowledgement in a paper can be "Achilles heel" for variety of reasons. The source of research funding, this should always be acknowledged, failure to do so is likely to constitute a violation of the condition. For example, sometimes within the published literature as a whole there can be certain extraordinary studies, which must have consumed resources that someone has paid for, and the author fails to mention this. Under such circumstances, the editor or the reader need to know the commercially interested body that has provided the resources, further this might raise a question whether the author is involved in a conflict of interest. Thus, acknowledgements should include contributors that need acknowledging but do not justify authorship. Authors should be those who can take full responsibility for the intellectual contents of the paper. On the other hand, individuals who have contributed to the originality of the work should be considered as coauthors.

An author can acknowledge anyone, e.g. a colleague, nurse and technician whose work has enabled the study to progress. In addition, individuals who have contributed intellectually to scientific paper can be listed with the description of contribution and function. For example, 'a scientific advisor', 'critical reviewer for study proposal', 'data collection' or 'participation in clinical trials' such contributors must give their permission to the author to have their name in the manuscript. In this respect, the author is also responsible for obtaining written permission from contributors to be acknowledged by name, because readers may infer their endorsement of the data and conclusions. The best way is to consult the contributor before the manuscript is sent for publication or the contributor should be made aware of who appears as a coauthor and who appears in acknowledgment section. At the same time, the acknowledgment section should not be seen as a 'catchall' for anyone you wish to flatter or do not wish to offend. Appearance of a name in acknowledgment implicate that the individual is held responsible if there is any controversy about the work once it is published. Moreover, the authors will be safe if there is appropriate consultation with the contributor before submission to the editor.

Recently, studies have been enrouted to develop automated intelligent methods for acknowledgement extraction and analysis to uncover important institutional and agency sponsors of scientific work. Analysis of financial support, instrumental/technical support in acknowledgment gives an insight into other trends in scientific communities, e.g. acknowledgment of financial support may be used to measure the relative impact of funding agencies and corporate sponsors on scientific research. Likewise acknowledgement of instrumental/technical support may be useful for analyzing indirect contributions of research laboratories and universities research activities. Through impact measures, it is made possible to compare the efficacy of funding agencies directly, because some funding programs may realize their impact in part by providing educational opportunities to young scientists rather than funding the best work in the field.

Added to these an author can recognize secretaries, wives or husbands, parents but not in the manuscripts. There have been occasions where the assistants have put more efforts in drafting the manuscript than the author; still it is not appropriate to mention their contribution in acknowledgment. Also, whom you choose to acknowledge can be impossible to separate from whom you choose to cite as an author on the byline. In this context, Vancouver group has specified a definite order of including the group members with their permission in acknowledgment:

1. Contribution that need acknowledging but do not justify authorship such as general support by departmental chair.
2. Acknowledgment of technical help.
3. Acknowledgment of financial and material support—specifying the nature of support.
4. Relationships that may pose a conflict of interest.

Always there is only one rule to bear in mind, when deciding who is an author, a contributor or an acknowledgee. Decide who is to be chosen as what before you start with the study. Many a time authorship disputes arise when the work is completed and the manuscript has to be written and sent for publication. Then comes the jostle for a position in the byline. Primary prevention is always better in the end.

SUGGESTED READING

1. Cronin B, McKenzie G, Rubio L, Weaver-Wozniak S. "Accounting for influence: acknowledgments in contemporary sociology." J *Am Soc Inform Sci* 1993; 44(7):406-12.
2. Cronin B, Shaw D, La Barre K. 'A cast of thousands' 'Co-authorship and sub-authorship collaboration in the twentieth century as manifested in the scholarly literature of psychology and philosophy'. J *Am Soc Inform Sci Technol* 2003;54(9): 855-71.
3. Edge D. Quantitative Measures of Communication in Science: A Critical Overview. Hist. Sci 1979;17:102-34.
4. Giles CL, Councill IG. Who gets acknowledged: measuring scientific contributions through automatic acknowledgment indexing. Proc Natl Acad Sci U S A. 2004;101(51):17599-604. Epub, 2004.
5. George M Hall (ed). How to write a paper 2nd Edn. Byword publisher Delhi, 2000.
6. Alastair A Spence (ed), How to write a paper 2nd edn. Delhi Byword Publisher, 2000.

18 Submitting the Manuscript

Fatema Jawad

INTRODUCTION

Research culminates in publication, which every author wishes to achieve. This desire is at times born even prior to submitting the manuscript to a journal. Before an article is finally sent for publication, many steps have to be taken which need hardwork, skill, time and perseverance. It is similar to sowing a seed, nurturing the plant till it grows to be a tree and finally gives the fruit.

It all begins with the scholar or researcher conceiving an idea, reading on the subject, performing the research, acquiring the results and finally comes the most crucial stage of getting it published. This can be made simple if the recommendations are followed.

The first step is to select a journal for submitting the article. Depending on the subject under study it could be a multidisciplinary journal or a subject specialized publication. It is advisable to select one or two journals before writing the research as it makes compliance to the guidelines easy.

To decide on an appropriate journal, the following points should be considered:

- Is the journal peer reviewed?
- Is the journal indexed with the major electronic databases as Medline, BIOSIS, Current Contents, etc.?
- How long has the journal being publishing? Established journals have a wider readership.
- What is the impact factor of the journal? Though not a very justified aspect, but it provides a good idea regarding the citation in the field.
- What is the frequency of publication, weekly, monthly, quarterly or bi-annual?
- What is the lag time for an article?

- Language of the journal. English language journals are more widely read.

To be accurate in conforming to the requirements of the selected journal, it is mandatory to read and again read the Guidelines to Authors for the selected journal. Most journals follow the "Uniform Requirements for Manuscripts submitted to Biomedical Journals," recommended by the International Committee of Medical Journal Editors (ICMJE) and available on its website, but each journal also has its own requirements along with the ICMJE guidelines. There can be a limitation on the length of the article in the form of word count for each section. Number of tables and figures can be specified and the maximum number of References for each category of article is usually stated.

Time management is an important aspect of submitting an article for publication. Making a schedule and following it is helpful. Every journal needs some time for processing a manuscript and it cannot be done in a hurry. The author should plan accordingly as a deadline for an examination is not a reason to speed up the process. If the time is short it will only spoil the author's nerves.

Coauthors should be justifiable. The coauthors are always decided upon before the article is written. It has to be like-minded colleagues who have contributed substantially to the research. Most journals ask for a detailed contribution of all authors and most standard journals follow the ICMJE Criteria for authorship.

1. Substantial contribution to research design, or the acquisition, analysis or interpretation of data.
2. Drafting the article or revising it critically for important intellectual content.
3. Final approval of the version to be published.

    Authors should meet all the three criteria.

COVER LETTER

This is the first to be read by the editor of a journal. It also forms the first impression of the authors. The letter should be brief with all the necessary information required which can be obtained from the website of the target journal.

The following points should be incorporated:

- Name, address, phone and fax numbers and email address of the corresponding author
- Alternative contact details in case of absence of the corresponding author

- A brief statement on the importance of the research done and why it should be published
- The originality of the work should be stated. If this article is part of a thesis or a larger study or has been presented in a conference, it should be clearly stated
- Any competing interest should be declared
- A certificate/declaration should be submitted to the effect that this manuscript has not been published or submitted for consideration of publication, in part or whole, to any other journal. This document has to be signed by all authors.

Sample Cover Letter (Used By JPMA) – Refer Box 18.1

Upon acceptance by Journal of the Pakistan Medical Association, all copyright ownership for the article is transferred to the Journal of Pakistan Medical Association.

Box 18.1: Sample Cover letter

We, the undersigned, principal author and coauthors of this article, have contributed significantly to and share in the responsibility for above. The undersigned stipulate that the material submitted to Journal of the Pakistan Medical Association is new, original and has not been submitted to another publication for concurrent consideration. It is also attested that neither this manuscript nor one with substantially similar contents has been published, submitted or is under consideration for publication.

The undersigned also declare that no unfair or unethical means have been employed to produce this manuscript and that no part of the submission has been plagiarized in any form. We also submit that we are aware of the JPMA Plagiarism Policy which we have read on the Journal website and are in total compliance with it.

We also attest that any human and /or animal studies undertaken as part of the research from which this manuscript was derived are in compliance with regulation of our institution(s) and with generally accepted guidelines governing such work.

We further attest that we have herein disclosed any and all financial or other relationships which could be construed as a conflict of interest and that all sources of financial support for this study have been disclosed and are indicated in the acknowledgement.

IMPORTANT CHECK POINTS BEFORE SUBMITTING A MANUSCRIPT

After the manuscript has been written and read by all authors, it should be put under a final scan of scrutinizing each section. The important check points for every section appear below.

Title: Is it informative and descriptive containing all the elements of the article? The title attracts readers so it is kept short and meaningful. Fancy titles are to be avoided.

Abstract: The abstract is a brief resume of the entire article. It is written after the article has been completed. It can be structured or unstructured in a paragraph form according to the requirements of the journal. The sequence has to be maintained. No references are given and no tables or figures referred. It is always written in the past tense.

Key Words: Existing key words are selected. Long ones are better avoided. Four to six words are sufficient.

Objective: A very precise objective should be stated giving the reason why the study was undertaken.

Background: The background is usually not necessary but if required a very brief introduction may be added.

Methods: This includes the design or type of study, setting or where was the study performed as Hospital/Community/Institutions and period of study. This is followed by patients/subjects/material, sample size and type, inclusion criteria, sociodemographic features, matching or control groups and follow-up.

Results: Relevant statistically analyzed results, both negative and positive are included. Tables and figures are not referred. Quantitative data is reported with statistical analysis results. The results should be the same as what is given in the main article.

Discussion: This is meant to interpret the study results. It should start with statement of principal findings followed by strength and weaknesses of the study. Detail results should not be repeated in the discussion section. Results may differ from other studies or agree with some research results. A comparison has to be made and the reasons for both discussed.

Conclusion: This should be brief and supporting the results.

INTRODUCTION: Refer Chapter 9 for details

The objective of this section is to introduce the subject, establish the context of the work being reported and give the importance of the study performed. It should justify the rationale of the study and why was the subject selected.

Introduction should be able to answer the following questions:
- What was I studying?
- What was known before the study?
- How will this study enhance our knowledge?
- Has the purpose of the study along with the scientific merits been stated?

The introduction should end with the objective of the study. The writing style is the past tense in simple, clear and using correct language. All important points should be stated in a paragraph form duly referenced, if other publications are quoted. Background information should be precise and with correct references.

METHODS: Refer Chapter 10 for details

Passive voice and third person in the past tense is recommended for writing this section.

What must be stated?

Type of study, location of study and period and duration of study.

Ethical Review Board's approval is mandatory and informed consent of the individuals studied. Both should be clearly stated. Inclusion and exclusion criteria and statistical tests applied are important aspects of the methods and should not be missed.

Technical information: If specific chemicals or apparatus have been used, the manufacturers name should be given with a reference. For well documented procedures the name is stated with a reference.

RESULTS: Refer Chapter 14 for details

Key findings have to be objectively presented. The demographic data is given in a sequence followed by the findings of the study which are stated in the text in order of relevance and in the context of the question addressed. After analysis of the data some results can be presented in a figure or table form. The details of each table or figure should not be written in the text format. They are referred as figure 1 or table 1. Raw data is not reported. Means and percentages are used. Important negative results should be included.

Figures and tables are numbered separately in a consecutive manner. The caption of the figure is written below and that of the table above. Each table and figure must provide complete information including standard deviations in mean values and p values for significance. Place each table and figure on a separate page.

DISCUSSION: Refer Chapter 15 for details

This is meant to interpret the study results. It is simple to write a structured discussion. It should start with statement of principal findings followed by strength and weaknesses of the study. Detail results should not be repeated in the discussion section. Results may differ from other studies or agree with some research results. A comparison has to be made and the reasons for both discussed. References are inserted where support is needed. If a new aspect of the subject has been identified which has proved as advancement to what is already known, it should be made evident. Strengths and weaknesses of the study have to be stated. Any alternative interpretations should be indicated. A new result discovered is always emphasized in the discussion. If there are any unanswered questions they should be included.

CONCLUSION

This highlights the results and goals of the study. A small paragraph, containing the final implications and applications. Recommendations are avoided. Comparisons are not made and no references are used.

ACKNOWLEDGEMENT: Refer Chapter 17 for details

All those who helped in the study should be acknowledged as colleagues who helped in designing the study but did not participate actively, physicians who referred cases, laboratory assistance, statisticians for statistical tests, secretarial help and outside reviewers for suggestions.

Any source of funding for supporting the research must be stated.

Any conflict of interest is always written.

REFERENCES: Refer Chapter 16 for details

Most journals follow the vancouver style. Six author's names are written before et al. Make sure that the references are placed in ascending order in the text and correspond with the numbers in the list.

GENERAL TIPS

Write in MS Word, 12 font and double spacing.

The first page should have the title of the article followed by the full names of the authors with their affiliations and address of institutions. The corresponding author's e-mail address and telephone number is mandatory.

The certificate of non-submission or copyright to the journal should be signed by all authors.

If the journal has the provision of online submission, follow the steps.

If the journal accepts articles via e-mail, send the completed document as an attachment along with a covering letter.

It is important to read the article multiple times by all authors to ensure that nothing is left out.

If all rules are followed, the article has a good chance of being accepted.

MODE OF SUBMISSION OF A MANUSCRIPT

- By mail (Post)
- Electronic submission—e-mail or online submission system and peer reviewing.

By Mail or Postage

This is not being used by most journals, in fact some journals clearly state in the instructions to authors that submission by mail is not acceptable. If permitted by the journal, then two hard copies should be prepared in double spacing, 12 point font size on MS Word. The digital version or soft copy should be placed as a CD. The authorship form and covering letter is attached to the manuscript. Mention type of submission in your cover letter with a word count.

Two sets of unmounted glossy Figures (no smaller than 3-1/2x5 inches and not larger than 8x10 inches) and the copyright transfer should be enclosed.

Title page should have the title, authors' names and complete affiliations; corresponding author's name and complete address, telephone number and e-mail address (necessary), author for reprint requests. All the documents are placed in a lined envelop and sent to the journal preferably by courier service.

Electronic Submission

E-mail submissions are in the form of attachments. The main manuscript is put in one folder. Photographs, graphs, tables and figures are prepared as separate attachments. The covering letter and authorship declaration is the third attachment. The signatures should be scanned, as without signatures, the document will not be accepted. Title page is the same providing the detail information of the authors.

Online Manuscript Submission

All the standard journals are using this system. The applicant is registered for an account and provided with a username and password which will be used for all times required. After logging in, the home page is reached which is personalized, listing different categories of tasks. Accurate commands are given to complete the process of submission. Articles should not be submitted as PDF format. Use Word or Word Perfect. Figures should be loaded as separate files, particularly for manuscripts with large numbers of figures. Most journals with the provision of online submission also have a tracking system for further enquiries. They also invite names of colleagues for peer review. The authors can suggest these to expedite the review process.

SUGGESTED READING

1. Docherty M, Smith R.The case for structuring the discussion of scientific papers. BMJ 1999;318:1224-5.
2. Uniform requirements for manuscripts submitted to biomedical journals: Writing and editing for biomedical publication. International committee of Medical Journal Editors. Available at www.icmje.org Cited 7. July, 2010.
3. Uniform requirements for manuscripts submitted to biomedical journals: Writing and editing for Biomedical publication. International committee of Medical Journal Editors. Available at www.icmje.org pp 2. Cited 7. July, 2010.

Section 4
Systematic review, Meta-analysis and Writing a non-research paper

19 Understanding Systematic Review and Meta-Analysis

Shailesh Lele

INTRODUCTION

One of the newer types of articles that we come across in biomedical journals is 'systematic review' or 'meta-analysis'. Traditional reviews are popular among authors for they are easier to prepare than conducting a trial. They are popular among readers because they make easy reading (sans the jargon and statistics) and provide a quick overview of the topic, especially to the harried students. With the evidence-based healthcare movement gaining ground, traditional reviews are not considered evidence for clinical effectiveness. The randomized, controlled clinical trials (RCTs) are the new blue-eyed boys in the hierarchy of evidence. However, one of the significant and frequent limitations of RCTs is small sample size, which may result in incorrect estimation of clinical effectiveness. Systematic reviews and meta-analyses, which summarize or combine several RCTs, therefore have emerged as the highest level of evidence in clinical practice (see Box 19.1). Also, the skills and time required to search and appraise research evidence may not be readily on hand to a clinician. Thus, therapy that is really beneficial to patients may not come in to practice, while therapy that is more harmful may continue to be practiced. In either case, patient is the loser! Systematic reviews provide evidence that could be readily applied in practice.

For long there has been a lamentation that the medical profession has failed to systematically summarize the evidence available in the numerous clinical trials. Archie Cochrane, from whose seminal work emerged evidence-based healthcare, wrote: "It is surely a great criticism of our profession that we have not organized a critical summary, by specialty or subspecialty, adapted periodically, of all relevant randomized controlled trials." Probably the first ever meta-analysis was prepared in 1904 by Karl Pearson—the statistician. Rediscovered in 1970s, scientific literature has seen an explosion of systematic reviews and meta-analyzes,

Box 19.1: Hierarchy of evidence
(Abridged from Oxford Center for Evidence-based Medicine)

Levels of evidence for effectiveness of therapy
1a	SR* of RCTs^
1b	Individual RCT^
1c	All or none
2a	SR* of cohort studies
2b	Individual cohort study
2c	Outcomes research; Ecological studies
3a	SR* of case-control studies
3b	Individual case-control study
4	Case-series
5	Expert opinion; Bench research

Grades of recommendation
A	Consistent level 1 studies
B	Consistent level 2 or 3 studies *or* extrapolations from level 1 studies
C	Level 4 studies *or* extrapolations from level 2 or 3 studies
D	Level 5 evidence *or* troublingly inconsistent or inconclusive studies of any level

*: Systematic Review, ^: Randomized controlled trial

especially in last couple of decades. PubMed identifies systematic reviews as a 'review' type of publication, while meta-analysis is a distinct publication type. In the period from 1948 to-date (28th June 2010), PubMed lists 1,523,555 review articles. In the same period, PubMed lists 20,906 articles with the phrase 'systematic review' either in the title or the abstract. It is interesting to note that only 67 of these were published prior to 1988. Again, of the remaining 20,839 articles as many as 9,118 were published in the last two and a half years alone (June 2008–2010). Since 1948 PubMed has indexed 24,651 articles as meta-analysis. More than 7,000 of these were published in the last two and a half years, while over 17,500 between 1988 and 2007. The Cochrane Collaboration (see Box 19.2) is in the forefront of this activity with thousands of systematic reviews in various stages of preparation, completion and updating under its aegis. Systematic reviews and meta-analyzes have also been accepted as scholarly works eligible for faculty appointments and promotions. It is estimated that at least 10,000 Cochrane Reviews are needed to cover all healthcare interventions that have already been investigated in controlled trials. Moreover, these reviews will need to be updated at the rate of 5000 per year. In this chapter, we shall see why these two types of works have evoked so much interest among researchers, academicians and healthcare providers, and how to prepare these types of reviews.

SYSTEMATIC REVIEW

In its glossary, Oxford Centre for Evidence-based Medicine describes a systematic review as "an article in which the authors have systematically searched for, appraised, and summarized all of the medical literature

Box 19.2: Cochrane Collaboration (from www.cochrane.org)

- International, independent, not-for-profit organization.
- Network of over 28,000 contributors from more than 100 countries.
- Primary activity is preparation, updating, dissemination, and promotion of systematic reviews.
- 53 Cochrane Review Groups in various health areas: e.g. Renal group, Skin group, Stroke group, Oral Health group.
- The Cochrane Library: an online collection of databases of rigorous and up-to-date research on the effectiveness of healthcare.
- Cochrane Database of Systematic Reviews (CDSR) contains over 4000 systematic reviews and over 2000 protocols (reviews in progress).
- CDSR 2009 impact factor: 5.653.
- Free access to users logging in from India to full reviews as well as other resources at http://www.thecochranelibrary.com.

for a specific topic". Besides being systematic, the methodology adapted for a systematic review is explicitly stated, and is therefore transparent and reproducible. The evidence from individual studies is not accepted at face value, but is critically examined for its validity and strength. The summary or the bottom line provides a definite guidance to the clinician, and may even synthesize new evidence. The Cochrane Collaboration describes a systematic review as an assembly of primary studies (predominantly RCTs), which are appraised for their research design and characteristics, their data synthesized and results interpreted. A comparison with the traditional literature review (also called a 'narrative review') would illustrate what a systematic review is.

Mostly, the narrative reviews lack focus and are compiled to provide an overview of a broad subject area. Sometimes, due to personal bias of the reviewer, only select literature is reviewed. Cates has given the analogy of the 'file-drawer problem': there is a natural tendency to collect in our desk drawer articles that fit in with our view and show the dustbin to the articles that do not. When asked to review a topic, it is natural then to go the drawer and quote all the data that supports our favorite view. Sufficient attempt may not be made to locate all the literature without any language or journal bias. Unpublished studies may go unnoticed. Convenience, rather than purposefulness, directs the search for studies. Further, in narrative reviews studies may not be critically examined ('appraisal') for correctness of research design and adherence to it. Conclusions from different studies are simply compiled. A conclusion of effectiveness of a therapy drawn from a case-control study would not be as valid as that drawn from a randomized controlled trial. A clinician is keen to know which intervention is going to work in a particular type of patient, and at what dosage and to what extent. Narrative reviews inform the clinician only about the various interventions available for a condition.

In 1972, Shaw reviewed the various modalities available then for investigating stroke patients. In the typical style of a narrative review, he first discusses classification of stroke. Next he reviews the investigations (viz. clinical history, radiography, EEG, brain scans, lumbar puncture and angiography) in patients with completed and other types of stroke. A Cochrane systematic review published in 2009 has estimated and compared the diagnostic accuracy of magnetic resonance imaging (MRI) for acute ischemic stroke with that of computed tomography (CT). Based on appraisal of eight studies, review authors conclude that MRI is more sensitive (0.99) than CT (0.39) while being comparable in specificity (0.92 and 1.00 respectively). Yet, they opine that the applicability of MRI in practice is limited due to its availability, cost and unsuitability in some stroke patients. Barnett has reviewed the progress made in stroke therapy in the past forty years. On the other hand, a Cochrane systematic review has specifically reviewed efficacy and safety of anti-platelet therapy in acute ischemic stroke. Based on the evidence from twelve trials, the authors conclude that oral aspirin (160-300 mg daily, started within 48 hours of onset) significantly reduces death or dependency (odds ratio - 0.95, NNT to benefit- 79).

Recommendations found in narrative reviews published in journals and textbooks often lag behind the systematic reviews by more than a decade in endorsing a treatment of proven effectiveness. They may continue to advocate a therapy long after it has been shown to be useless or even harmful. One glaring example concerns use of beta blockers after myocardial infarction. Many RCTs were available on this issue since 1967. A systematic review of these trials prepared in 1981 calculated 20% reduction in mortality with use of beta blockers. Yet, till 1989 medicine textbooks did not advocate their use.

This comparison is not to deride the narrative review (it does serve a purpose, albeit different), but to highlight how a systematic review differs from it (see Box 19.3). As could be seen in the comparison, a systematic review informs the clinician in making a decision on investigation or therapy. In more ways than one, preparing a systematic review is like conducting a clinical trial. The difference being that in a systematic review, the 'subjects' are the clinical trials themselves. Just like a clinical trial, there is an objective and stated methodology ('protocol'); inclusion of trials based on pre-defined criteria (mostly published reports of RCTs, but unpublished trials are also eligible); appraising the trials in an un-biased manner; synthesis of results; and conclusions based on the evidence.

Advantages of Systematic Reviews

The comparison made in the previous section brings out several advantages that systematic reviews have over the narrative reviews and other types of literature.

	Box 19.3: Narrative versus Systematic Review	
Feature	*Narrative Review*	*Systematic Review*
• Scope	• Usually covers broad topic area	• Addresses a focused clinical question.
• Method	• Not explicit	• Systematic, explicit and reproducible.
• Sources	• Usually limited to articles that support reviewer's views	• Attempts to locate all published articles and even data from unpublished trials.
• Search	• Does not have a pre-determined strategy	• Uses explicit search strategy that specifies the sources to be searched, publication years, and the type of studies to be looked for.
• Selection of studies	• Does not specify criteria. All types of articles may be reviewed	• Adheres to pre-determined inclusion criteria: type of study and rigor of study design • Reviewers are often blinded to authorship and source journal.
• Appraisal	• Usually no appraisal. Only the study conclusions are compiled	• Data from included studies is extracted to pre-designed forms. • Variable weightage is given to data from different quality studies.
• Synthesis	• It is a qualitative summary.	• It is often supplemented by quantitative summary ("meta-analysis")
• Conclusions	• Mostly ends with topic status or trends.	• Its bottom-line is evidence-based.
• Application	• Mostly academic since even animal or laboratory studies may be included. • Useful in understanding basic physiology and pathology. • Most useful for obtaining a broad perspective on a topic. • Provides directions for future research.	• Informs in making clinical decisions since only scientifically valid trials in human are included. • Useful in healthcare policy and administration, medico-legal issues, and health insurance. • Helps in defining current standards of healthcare based on science. • Cochrane reviews provide summaries for consumers, and support and advocacy groups. • Preparing a review trains the authors in critical appraisal skills.
• Authors	• Usually one-person effort	• More than one reviewer involved at every stage of review. • Supported by several others.
• Peer review	• Usually not.	• At every stage.
• Update	• May not be done	• Mandatory for Cochrane reviews every year or two.

1. The explicit, pre-determined methodology for searching and selecting studies limits bias and random error.
2. Combining studies makes conclusions more reliable and accurate.
3. More information is obtained ('synthesis') from existing data. Benefits or hazards not apparent in small studies could be detected.
4. A large amount of information from several studies becomes available in a processed format that is suitable for healthcare providers, researchers, policymakers and consumers.
5. The gap between research findings and implementation of effective diagnostic and therapeutic strategies or discontinuation of ineffective or harmful strategies may be reduced.
6. If results of different studies are consistent, it becomes possible to generalize them. If conclusions are valid and strong, further research could be halted to save resources.
7. If results of different studies are inconsistent, it may generate new hypotheses that could be tested in future research.
8. Preparing a systematic review is a scholarly exercise, which makes the reviewer conversant with research methodology, biostatistics, and systematic searching of databases and journals. It also helps develop critical appraisal skills in the reviewer.
9. Systematic reviews can enhance training, especially postgraduate, in several ways.

Limitations of Systematic Reviews

There are certain inherent limitations of systematic reviews.
1. The attribute of being focused may itself be a limitation while applying the conclusions to a clinical situation.
2. Ironically, there is limited evidence on whether applying systematic review conclusions (or for that matter evidence-based medicine) in practice leads to better healthcare for patients.
3. There is some doubt whether conclusions of effectiveness derived from data on a patient cohort would be applicable to an individual patient.
4. At least two good quality RCTs are needed to prepare a systematic review.
5. Bias and methodological errors occur in systematic reviews just as they do in narrative reviews. Different systematic reviews on the same topic may produce conflicting conclusions.
6. A therapy found effective in a systematic review may increase healthcare costs, or may not be acceptable to a patient, or healthcare provider may not possess the skills needed to implement it.
7. Unless regularly updated to include new studies, systematic reviews quickly get outdated.

8. Systematic review is but one of the inputs in making clinical decisions. It can aid but not replace a clinician's expertise, who understands the patient's circumstances, expectations and values in totality.

Preparing a Systematic Review

We are all aware how difficult it is to stay up-to-date with literature. Locating new studies, and reading and assimilating them are daunting tasks. One needs to go beyond these steps in preparing a high-quality systematic review. Yet, having prepared one, the satisfaction is rewarding, especially if it significantly impacts practice.

The basic format for a systematic review is fairly standard: one begins by identifying the problem area; formulates a hypothesis or a focused question; outlines the methods for searching, selecting and appraising studies; synthesizes the results of included studies; and provides a clinically useful bottom-line. While one could independently prepare a systematic review, it is recommended that it is prepared under the auspices of the Cochrane Collaboration. The guidance, support, resources and the network of highly-motivated reviewers not only makes the task little less demanding, but also ensures review quality. Further, the Cochrane Collaboration is committed to disseminate the reviews worldwide, thus assuring much wider impact. The stages in preparing a review are depicted in Figure 19.1 and described below.

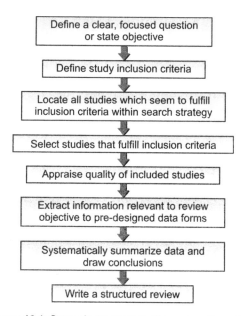

Figure 19.1: Stages in preparation of a systematic review

Define a Clear, Focused Question/State objective

At the end of a busy day in the clinic, you often wonder whether some of the patients could have been treated in a better way. A new drug therapy introduced by manufacturer's representative seemed to have potential to work in patients. The representative gave you several citations claiming superiority of this new therapy. Looking up their abstracts, you are still not clear about its effectiveness. Questions start forming in your mind: would this new therapy work in the type of patients in my practice, and to what extent when compared to current therapy? Would there be any harmful effects? This could be the genesis of a systematic review. However, in order to get clinically applicable conclusive answers, these questions need to be focused. PICO format is recognized as a standard format to define review question.

P: Patient or population or problem

I: Intervention you are curious about

C: Comparison with the currently used therapy or with placebo or no therapy

O: Outcomes that you hope to see in patients

For example

- In hypertensive patients, would the use of angiotensin receptor blocker when compared to placebo/ currently used drug affect (increase/ decrease) risk of myocardial infarction?
- In patients with osteoarthritis, is intra-articular corticosteroid injection when compared to placebo/ other corticosteroid therapies effective in improving symptoms/ range of joint movement/ harmful to the joint?
- In patients with furcation periodontitis, would guided tissue regeneration when compared to standard surgical debridement reduce open horizontal furcation depth?

Alternatively, question could be rephrased and stated as the review objective. For example:

- To evaluate the effect of angiotensin receptor blockers on the risk of myocardial infarction in patients at risk for cardiovascular events
- To determine the efficacy of intra-articular corticosteroid injections for osteoarthritis of the knee and to identify numbers needed to treat
- To systematically review the evidence of effectiveness of guided tissue regeneration (GTR) for furcation defects.

Not only does such clear language make the question answerable, it also assists greatly in locating every potentially relevant study in the literature (see below). It also defines the scope of the review and enhances its potential to aid clinical decision-making. As the time and resources to answer a plethora of questions are limited, reviewers must choose the most important questions. The personal curiosity of the reviewer notwithstanding, questions that deal with conditions that have a major effect on patients or on persons who care for them or on the whole community should be posed. Majority of interventions have potentially harmful effects, and these should be evaluated in the review.

Define Study Inclusion Criteria

It is obvious that only those studies that address the four components in the PICO format should be included in the review. However, it is still necessary to define beforehand specific criteria for each component. In other words, each component needs to be expanded. Patient or problem characteristics may be defined in terms of gender, age, disease duration or intensity, setting in which the therapy is to be instituted, concomitant conditions, etc. Similarly the intervention of interest should be described in terms of dosage, duration and route of administration.

To evaluate true effectiveness of a therapy, it needs to be compared with no treatment or placebo administration. However, ethical considerations may not allow this comparison. Therefore, in most clinical trials control comparison is with active treatment. A variety of outcomes are assessed by different researchers. Outcomes of patients' interest are: increased survival, reduced morbidity, reduction in symptoms, improved function, better quality of life, no harmful effects, and economy. A clinician may also be interested in resolution of lesion, and biochemical or histological indicators. Although only RCTs should be included in systematic reviews, not every RCT may have adhered to the rigor expected in it. For example: patient allocation may be quasi-randomized and may not be concealed, outcome assessment may not be blinded, other than the intervention the trial groups may not have been equally treated, or loss of patients to follow-up may not be taken in to analysis.

Finally, it is always a balancing act between how broad or narrow the inclusion criteria should be. Too narrow criteria may leave very few studies for the review, which even while providing more precise estimates of effectiveness, is less generalisable. Since, systematic review methods allow weighted estimates based on study quality, it may be wiser to err on the broader side. An initial survey of literature provides clues about the characteristics of clinical trials available in the literature. If due cognizance of these is taken, a clear and focused question and a set of inclusion criteria would emerge. A strong foundation would be laid to build a high-quality review.

The inclusion criteria in the earlier cited Cochrane systematic review on anti-platelet therapy is an excellent example of well-defined criteria. An abridged version is reproduced below:

- Participants: Patients of any age or sex within two weeks of onset of presumed ischemic stroke
- Intervention: Either a single anti-platelet agent or a combination of anti-platelet agents
- Comparison: With control (placebo or no treatment)
- Outcomes: Number of participants who were either dead, or dependent on help from other people for their activities of daily living, at least one month after their stroke

Locate all Studies which Seem to Fulfill Inclusion Criteria with Search Strategy

A systematic review is expected to summarize results of all the studies relevant to the review objective. Study results are available in a variety of sources: journals; conference proceedings; books; reference lists; trial registries; manufacturers' records; electronic databases; unpublished studies; personal communications; and thesis and dissertations submitted to universities. A comprehensive search strategy is required to locate as many of them as the resources allow minimizing bias and random error.

The inclusion criteria guide the search process. The terms and phrases defined in the expanded PICO format form the basis of this process. The electronic databases (both the general like MEDLINE, Embase and subject-specific like CINAHL, CANCERLIT) are the major source to locate studies. Searching these databases for studies potentially relevant to the review objective is a new skill that a reviewer needs to acquire and master. A basic understanding of indexing process, standard terminologies (e.g. MeSH in MEDLINE) and search methods specific to a database are essential for an efficient and comprehensive search. Fortunately, every database provides a set of tools that make the process a little easier. For example: the 'Limits' option in PubMed allows one to locate studies carried out in a specific gender or age group. It also categorizes studies based on the design; like clinical trial, randomized controlled trial, and case series. Yet, it must be remembered that indexing is done by humans and is as much prone to error as any other human activity. Therefore, very elaborate search strategies specific to a database have been developed. These follow the funnel principle: the initial search is very sensitive to identify every possible study; this is followed by strategies that step-by-step eliminate most of the irrelevant studies. Still the reviewer may be left with about hundred potentially relevant studies, which need to be individually scanned for possible inclusion. An example of highly sensitive search filter to identify controlled trials in PubMed is reproduced in Box 19.4. Cochrane Collaboration review groups have also developed specific search strategies. Niederman and others have developed MEDLINE search strategies to locate RCTs in seven dental disciplines.

Box 19.4: Cochrane highly sensitive search filter to identify controlled trials

(randomized controlled trial[pt] OR controlled clinical trial[pt] OR randomized controlled trials[mh] OR random allocation[mh] OR double-blind method[mh] OR single-blind method[mh] OR clinical trial[pt] OR clinical trials[mh] OR ("clinical trial"[tw]) OR ((singl*[tw] OR doubl*[tw] OR trebl*[tw] OR tripl*[tw]) AND (mask*[tw] OR blind*[tw])) OR ("latin square"[tw]) OR placebos[mh] OR placebo*[tw] OR random*[tw] OR research design[mh:noexp] OR comparative study[mh] OR evaluation studies[mh] OR follow-up studies[mh] OR prospective studies[mh] OR cross-over studies[mh] OR control*[tw] OR prospectiv*[tw] OR volunteer*[tw]) NOT (animal[mh] NOT human[mh])

Besides searching the electronic databases, other approaches are required to make the search really all-inclusive. These are:

- Hand-searching of relevant journals
- Tracking studies from the reference lists of published articles, other reviews, practice guidelines and government reports
- Looking-up clinical trial registries and conference proceedings
- Correspondence with manufacturers, subject experts, colleagues, authors of published studies, special interest groups and patient-support groups.

These approaches are very demanding in terms of diligence and time. Once the search exercise is complete, citations of all the potentially relevant studies should be exported to reference manager software (such as EndNote: www.endnote.com).

Select Studies that Fulfill Inclusion Criteria

Once the potentially relevant studies have been located, the inclusion criteria are applied to each study by two reviewers. To minimize bias, it is advisable to mask the author and publication information, and that one of the reviewers is a non-expert. Using a checklist of inclusion criteria, each reviewer independently scrutinizes the title and abstract (if available) of every study. Studies that seem to fulfill the inclusion criteria are selected; the remaining rejected. Disagreement between two reviewers is sorted out through discussion or in some instances by a third reviewer. This then becomes the final set of studies included in the review. The entire process is documented, especially reasons for rejecting a study.

Appraise Quality of Included Studies

The chief purpose of a systematic review is to summarize the evidence on a specific clinical question. One of the secondary objectives is to appraise the quality of the primary studies. If results across studies are at variance with each other (heterogeneity), the reasons are explored. Appraisal of study quality not only ascertains its internal validity, but also indicates its external validity (applicability to patients outside the study).

The full papers of the included studies are obtained for quality appraisal and data extraction. Again, two reviewers undertake this exercise independently. The study design decides the criteria for quality assessment. For example: criteria for an RCT could be concealed allocation of treatment, blinding of clinicians and outcome assessors, and information on reasons for withdrawal from trial group. The studies are also assessed for intention to treat analysis, comparability of groups at baseline, withdrawals, and whether other treatments (excluding those to which the patients were randomized) could have biased the results. While assessing quality, it is helpful to remember that there is often a gap between doing an RCT and reporting it. Some of these criteria for quality assessment may not have been reported. In such instances, it is prudent to contact the study authors to obtain missing information. The appraised studies may be graded for quality, and low-quality studies may be excluded from the review. Detailed tables are prepared summarizing characteristics of included and excluded studies.

Extract Information Relevant to Review Objective to Pre-designed Data Forms

Quality assessment and data extraction are usually done simultaneously using pre-designed data forms. Information is extracted on study characteristics, methodology, population characteristics, interventions and outcomes (including adverse effects). A look at the published systematic reviews and other resources would provide good guidance to build these forms. Since the entire analysis and conclusion shall emanate from the data extracted from the primary studies, ample time and thought should be invested in their designs. The form design should be pilot-tested on few representative studies and revised, if needed. Similar to the previous two stages, data extraction should also be done by two reviewers independently. This stage in the systematic review also serves to verify study eligibility.

Systematically Summarize Data and Draw Conclusions

To make sense of the extracted data, summary tables are prepared on the treatment effects obtained in all the studies. These are constructed for each outcome (including adverse effects), grouping together studies that are similar in terms of design, disease characteristics, intervention and length of follow-up. Treatment effects are usually expressed as risk ratios, odds ratios or difference between means for continuous outcomes. Numbers needed to treat (NNT) or harm (NNH) is another expression of clinical significance. Systematic reviews of diagnostic studies usually express outcomes in terms of sensitivity and specificity.

Forest plots provide a convenient visual summary of effects. For illustration purpose, a forest plot from a fictional systematic review is reproduced in Figure 19.2. Other graphs include funnel plot and L'Abbé plot. Overall patterns, correlations and outlying observations that might otherwise be overlooked could be identified in graphs. Possible trends may also emerge in a graph. Graphs save the reader considerable time and effort in absorbing the findings of a systematic review, and can facilitate comparison of data across different scenarios.

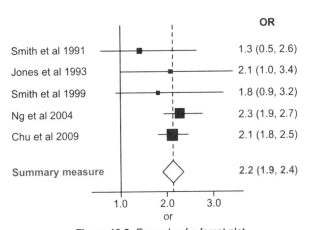

Figure 19.2: Example of a forest plot
Odds ratio with confidence interval of each study is represented by a solid square and horizontal line passing through it. Square size is proportional to weight assigned to the study. Overall effectiveness is represented by the centre line of diamond and associated confidence intervals by the lateral tips of diamond. Solid vertical line represents no effect (1.0)

Variability in patient characteristics, interventions and outcomes (clinical heterogeneity) or in study design (methodological heterogeneity) affects the treatment effects. Such heterogeneity in studies may warrant sub-group analysis of results. While this exercise does not affect the internal validity of studies, it precludes drawing overall single conclusion thus reducing its external validity (applicability). Sensitivity analysis gives a good indication of the robustness of the review methodology. This analysis ascertains impact of changing some of the parameters used (inclusion criteria, including studies that were excluded, statistical approach) in summarizing the results on treatment effects. If the sensitivity analyses that are done do not materially change the results, it strengthens the confidence that can be placed in these results. If the results do change in a way that might lead to different conclusions, this indicates a need for greater caution in interpreting the results and drawing conclusions.

The systematic review process concludes by interpreting the results. Primary purpose of the review is to inform the reader, and not to offer advice. The conclusions should present the evidence in an unambiguous manner, which could be used as one of the inputs while making clinical decisions. Applicability of conclusions should have an international perspective, and not restrict to national or local circumstances. Users of systematic reviews are interested in applicability of review conclusions to their patients. Review conclusions should therefore revolve around the strength of evidence.

Treatment effectiveness is essentially establishing a cause-and-effect relationship between the intervention and the outcomes. Hill's guidelines to establish this relationship require that the reviewer clearly states the following in the review conclusions:

- Circumstances (patient and disease characteristics, intervention) under which the treatment effects could be obtained
- Limitations of the review itself
- Quality level of the studies
- Size and significance of effects and their consistency across studies
- Dose-response relationship
- Indirect evidence (biological, animal studies) that supports the observed effects.

Such conclusions reflect strength of evidence and considerably enhance the applicability of review results. This could be further enhanced by information on harms and costs of the intervention when compared with the current practice. Similar to any research exercise, systematic review conclusions should be derived from the data extracted from the included studies. Temptation to broaden the conclusions beyond the limits set by the focused question should be resisted.

Write a Structured Review

Before launching in to the actual review process, it is advisable to prepare a synopsis consisting of the title; review background; question/objective; and detailed methodology for searching, appraising and summarizing studies. This synopsis should be improved after going through peer review process. If you are planning a Cochrane review, writing such synopsis (called a 'protocol') and its peer review is mandatory. Reading the protocols published in the Cochrane Library is quite educative.

If you intend to publish the review, guidelines on how to structure such reviews provided by the target journal should be followed. These are mostly similar to those for reporting original research (IMRaD format). However, considering that preparing a systematic review is an intricate task requiring a multitude of skills and that it requires substantial resources and support from several individuals, it is advisable to register a topic ('title') with one of the Cochrane Collaboration review groups. The review group and the wider collaboration provide all the resources, including human, at every stage of review preparation. All the resources are available free and the review is disseminated to an international audience.

The structure of a Cochrane review is given in Box 19.5. Another valuable resource—Cochrane Handbook for Systematic Reviews of Interventions—besides taking you through the entire review process also guides in writing the review. Berkeley Systematic Reviews Group (www.medepi.org/meta) and Center for Reviews and Dissemination (www.york.ac.uk/inst/crd) are also excellent resources for reviewers.

Box 19.5: Structure of a Cochrane systematic review

- Cover page
- Title
- Reviewers' information, Citation, Copyright
- Abstract: Background, Objectives, Search strategy, Selection criteria, Data collection and analysis, Main results, Authors' conclusion
- Plain language summary (for public)
- Main text: Background, Objectives, Methods, Results, Discussion, Authors' conclusions, Acknowledgements, Contribution of authors, Declaration of interests, Differences between protocol and review, Published notes
- Tables
- Studies and references
- Data and analyzes
- Figures
- Sources of support
- Appendices

META-ANALYSIS

When a systematic review uses statistical methods to combine and summarize the results of several primary studies, it is termed as 'meta-analysis' (therefore also called as 'quantitative systemic review'). As the name suggests, it goes beyond the data analyses done in the review.

Standardization of study designs is making it more and more possible to formally combine data from several studies with similar characteristics. While for binary (dichotomous) outcomes the results of meta-analysis are presented as measure of risk, for continuous variables the results are presented as weighted mean difference for the effect. Confidence intervals (95%) provide the precision of the estimate. Summary values calculated for each study are assigned weighting based on the study's precision. These are then combined and presented as a summary value, 95% confidence interval and P-value for the effect.

Besides the Review Manager, there are several other softwares available for conducting meta-analysis. While some need to be purchased (Stata, SAS, MetaWin), Meta-DiSc is a free package specifically designed for diagnostic meta-analysis. QUORUM guidelines are used to report a meta-analysis.

SUMMARY

In this chapter, salient features of systematic reviews and meta-analyzes have been presented along with a more detailed description of how to prepare a systematic review. While systematic reviews of RCTs are at the pinnacle of hierarchy of evidence, reviews of other types of studies (cohort, case-control and even single patient data) could also be prepared. These form the next link in the chain of 'next-best evidence'. While majority of systematic reviews are of intervention studies, reviews are also prepared of etiology, diagnosis, prevention, prognosis and economic studies. It seems logical that such reviews and meta-analyses would change the clinical practice for more benefits and less harm to patients. There is some evidence that it is indeed the case.

It is hoped that this chapter would be a sufficient practical guide to get started on systematic review preparation. It would be even more satisfying if it kindles interest among clinicians and researchers to take up the challenge of preparing systematic reviews in their areas of healthcare. These reviews would bridge the gap between research and practice, and point out areas where more research is needed. Benefit to patients may be maximized while minimizing the harm. Thus, in the final analysis, patient would emerge the winner!

SUGGESTED READING

1. Arroll B, Goodyear-Smith F. Corticosteroid injections for osteoarthritis of the knee: meta-analysis. BMJ, doi:10.1136/bmj.38039.573970.7C (published 23 March 2004).
2. Barnett HJM. Forty years of progress in stroke. Stroke 2010; 41:1068.
3. Berkeley Systematic Reviews Group. http://www.medepi.net/meta/forms.html. Accessed on 16th July 2010.

4. Brazzelli M, Sandercock PAG, Chappell FM, Celani MG, Righetti E, Arestis N, Wardlaw JM, Deeks JJ. Magnetic resonance imaging versus computed tomography for detection of acute vascular lesions in patients presenting with stroke symptoms. Cochrane Database of Systematic Reviews 2009, Issue 4.

5. Briffa T, Hickling S, Knuiman M, Hobbs M, Hung J, Sanfilippo FM, Jamrozik K, Thompson PL. Long term survival after evidence based treatment of acute myocardial infarction and revascularisation: follow-up of population based Perth MONICA cohort, 1984-2005. BMJ 2009;338:b36 (Published 26 January 2009).

6. Cates C. http://www.nntonline.net/ebm/newsletter/2003/10/Systematic_ Reviews_and _Meta-analyses.asp. Accessed on 28th June 2010.

7. Chung M, Balk EM, Brendel M, Ip S, Lau J, Lee J, Lichtenstein A, Patel K, Raman G, Tatsioni A, Terasawa T, Trikalinos TA. Vitamin D and calcium: A systematic review of health outcomes. http://www.ncbi.nlm.nih.gov/ bookshelf/picrender.fcgi? Book=erta183&blobtype=pdf. Downloaded on 16th July 2010.

8. Cook DJ, Mulrow CD, Haynes RB. Synthesis of best evidence for clinical decisions. Ann Intern Med 1997;126:376-80.

9. Counsell C. Formulating questions and locating primary studies for inclusion in systematic reviews. Ann Intern Med 1997;127:380-7.

10. Crombie IK, Davies HT. What is meta-analysis? Evidence-based Medicine. What is...? series. 2nd edition (2009). www.whatisseries.co.uk.

11. Egger M, Smith GD, Altman DG (eds). Systematic reviews in health care. Meta-analysis in context. London:BMJ Publishing Group 2001; pp. 3-19.

12. Egger M, Smith GD. Meta-analysis: Potentials and promise. BMJ 1997; 315:1371-4.

13. Higgins JPT, Green S, editors. Cochrane handbook for systematic reviews of interventions 4.2.6 [updated September 2006]. http://www.cochrane.org/ resources/ handbook/hbook.htm. Accessed on 26th June 2010.

14. Hill AB. The environment and disease: association or causation? Proc R Soc Med 1965;58:295-300.

15. James Lind Library. http://www.jameslindlibrary.org/trial_records/ 20th_Century/ 1940s/cochrane/cochrane_biog.html. Accessed on 28th June 2010.

16. Jepsen S, Eberhard J, Herrera D, Needleman I. A systematic review of guided tissue regeneration for periodontal furcation defects. What is the effect of guided tissue regeneration compared with surgical debridement in the treatment of furcation defects? J Clin Periodontol 2002;29(3):103-16.

17. Lele S, Hooper L. Pharmacological interventions for pain in patients with temporomandibular disorders (TMD). http://www.mrw.interscience. wiley.com/cochrane/clsysrev/articles/CD004715/pdf_fs.html.

18. McDonald MA, Simpson SH, Ezekowitz JA, Gyenes G, Tsuyuki RT. Angiotensin receptor blockers and risk of myocardial infarction: systematic review. BMJ, doi:10.1136/bmj.38595.518542.3A (published 29 September 2005).

19. Needleman I. A guide to systematic reviews. J Clin Periodontol 2002;29 (3):6-9.

20. Niederman R, Chen L, Murzyn L, Conway S. Benchmarking the dental randomized controlled literature on MEDLINE. Evidence-Based Dentistry 2002;3:5-9.

21. Oxford Centre for Evidence-based Medicine. http://www.cebm.cebm.neto= 1116. Accessed on 28th June 2010.

22. Oxford Centre for Evidence-based Medicine. http://www.cebm.netindex.aspxo =1025. Accessed on 28th June 2010.

23. Pai M, Mcculloch M, Gorman JD, Pai N, Enanoria W, Kennedy G, Tharyan P, Colford JM. Systematic reviews and meta-analyses: An illustrated, step-by-step guide. Natl Med J India 2004;17:86-95.

24. Sandercock PAG, Counsell C, Gubitz GJ, Tseng MC. Antiplatelet therapy for acute ischemic stroke. Cochrane Database of Systematic Reviews 2008, Issue 3.

25. Shaw DA. Investigation of stroke. BMJ 1972;1:91-3.

26. University of Washington Medicine. http://uwmedicine.washington.edu/ Global/ policies/ Pages/ Faculty-Appointments-and-Promotion-Guide.aspx. Accessed on 28th June 2010.

27. What are Cochrane reviews? The Cochrane Collaboration. http://www.cochrane.org/cochrane-reviews. Accessed on 28th June 2010.

28. "Wikimedia" http://upload.wikimedia.org/wikipedia/commons/f/f0/Generic forest_plot.png.http://upload.wikimedia.org/wikipedia/commons/f/f0/ Generic_forest_plot.png. Accessed on 19th July 2010.

20 How to Write an Invited Review Paper?*

INTRODUCTION

An invited review, also known as a review article, consists of a detailed and comprehensive narrative analysis of recent or evolving developments in a specific topic. It serves to highlight important points that have been previously reported in the literature. Unlike an original article, this type of paper does not introduce new information, and unlike an invited commentary, it does not include the author's opinion or personal experience. Invited articles are also different from systematic reviews.

Invited reviews are often favored by journal stakeholders. From the editor's perspective, reviews are often the most widely read articles in journals and are likely to be cited. For readers, invited reviews provide a good update of a particular topic and are a convenient way of keeping a practicing clinician or researcher current. For the author, being invited to contribute an invited review is usually regarded as a distinct honor. As its name implies, reviews are usually invited by the editor. Authors who are invited to provide a review article are acknowledged to have a particular expertise and extensive experience in that field. The authors are expected to provide a balanced article that puts the topic under discussion into the appropriate clinical and research perspective. Therefore, most authors would readily accept such an invitation. As these individuals often have heavy commitments, it is not unusual for them, ideally with the agreement of the editor, to act as senior authors and give the opportunity to a junior colleague to be the lead author in writing the manuscript for an invited review. Some journals do not accept unsolicited reviews, while others would consider such submissions and perhaps subject them to a more rigorous peer review. Generally, unsolicited

* Reproduced with permission - Peh W C G, Ng K H, Writing an invited review, Singapore Med J 2010; 51(4) : 271

reviews are much less likely to be accepted compared to invited ones. For authors who wish to write an unsolicited review, it is advisable to contact the journal editor ahead of time with the proposed topic and content outline. The editor's preliminary response should give the author an idea of whether or not to proceed, and hence save the author from wasted time, effort and potential disappointment. As invited reviews are one of the many types of articles that appear in medical journals, authors need to be aware of the specific requirements for their preparation. Most general medical and specialty journals do publish invited reviews, with their exact numbers being dependent on the vision of the editor and the mission of that particular journal. Several journals publish only invited reviews, such as the "Seminars", "Critical Reviews" and "Clinics of North America" series. Similar to all other manuscript types, the submitted manuscript for an invited review should also be constructed exactly according to the prescribed guidelines set by the target journal, which can usually be found in the journal's instructions to Authors. The authors should also be familiar with the journal readership, so that the invited review is tailored for the target audience.

STRUCTURE AND CONTENTS OF AN INVITED REVIEW (BOX 20.1)

Invited reviews should consist of the following headings: Unstructured abstract, introduction, subheadings to organize the topic in a logical manner, and a summary. Unlike original articles, invited reviews do not follow the IMRAD structure of manuscript organization.[1] In preparing to write an invited review, it is good practice to begin by making an outline comprising the major topic subheadings. This outline may possibly be shown to the editor, and then modified and further refined following discussion and mutual agreement. For some journals, such an outline is published as a "table of contents" for the invited review.

Box 20.1: Structure of an invited review

- Title
- Unstructured abstract
- Introduction
- Subheadings to organize material
- Summary
- References (extensive number)
- Illustrations (limited number)

A provisional title would often have been provided by the journal editor who has invited the review. If the author is unhappy with the title provided, he could ask for it to be altered.[2] Generally, titles should be as concise as possible, and yet clearly convey the main purpose of the review. Sometimes, a provocative title, perhaps posed as a question, would attract wider readership, particularly if the topic is debatable or controversial.[3] Some examples of invited review titles published in the Singapore Medical Journal over the past 15 months include:

- The anesthetist's role in the setting up of an intraoperative MR imaging facility
- Impact of the impact factor in biomedical research: its use and misuse
- Human bone marrow-derived adult stem cells for post-myocardial infarction cardiac repair: current status and future directions
- Pathological examination of the placenta: *Raison d'être*, clinical relevance and medicolegal utility
- Diagnosis and endoscopic resection of early gastric cancer

An unstructured abstract serves to provide a brief overview of the topic and conclusions. This is usually best written last, when the manuscript has been completed. It should be a clear and succinct summary of the important points and conclusions in the review. Abstracts for invited reviews typically consist of 75 to 300 words. In contrast to other paper categories, the main text of an invited review is usually relatively long, and should follow a prescribed word limit, typically up to 15 manuscript pages or up to 4,000 words, with variations according to the individual journal's Instructions to Authors. The introduction often includes the historical context of the topic and explains why the topic is important in current clinical or scientific practice. This aims to provide the background to the main body of the review which is to follow. The main body of a review is usually organized into subheadings, which varies according to the nature of the topics being reviewed. Conventionally, subheadings for a clinical review paper may include etiology, pathogenesis, clinical manifestations, investigative findings (including imaging and pathology), treatment and prognosis. Details of a specific procedure (e.g. indications, selection of appropriate patients, execution, complications), features of a specific condition, or strengths and weaknesses of the use of techniques, may be included (Box 20.2).

Box 20.2: Examples of subheadings for the main text of invited reviews:

Example 1
Title: Artifacts in musculoskeletal magnetic resonance imaging: identification and correction
[Authored by Peh WCG, Chan JHM. Published in Skeletal Radiology 2001; 30:179-91].
Subheadings:
- Introduction
- Motion artifacts
- Protocol-error artifacts

Contd...

Contd...
- Truncation artifacts
- Chemical shift artifacts
- Susceptibility artifacts
- Special artifacts
- Summary

Example 2
Title: Primary bone tumors of adulthood [Authored by Teo HEL, Peh WCG. Published in Cancer Imaging 2004; 4:74-83].
Subheadings:
- Introduction
- Imaging techniques
  - Radiography
  - CT
  - MR imaging
  - Bone scintigraphy
  - Image-guided biopsy
- Specific tumors by age
  - 20–30 years
  - 30–50 years
  - > 50 years
Staging
  - Surgical stage of bone tumors
  - Grade
  - Site
  - Metastasis
  - Staging and limb salvage surgery
- Conclusion

Example 3
Title: Image-guided musculoskeletal biopsy [Authored by Gogna A, Peh WCG, Munk PL. Published in Radiologic Clinics of North America 2008; 46:455-73].
Subheadings:
- Introduction
- Preparation
  - Why must one perform this biopsy?
  - Indications and contraindications
  - Percutaneous or open biopsy?
  - When is it safe and appropriate to proceed?
- Technique and equipment
  - Preliminary preparation
  - Positioning
  - Route
  - Types of lesions/lesion characteristics
  - Needle types
  - Techniques
  - Does size matter?
  - Image guidance modality and biopsy techniques
  - Handling of specimens
  - Tips for successful biopsy
  - Expected results
  - Post procedure routine
  - Complications
- Summary

The author should have critically assessed the available evidence. Papers that do not provide sufficiently useful information or evidence should be rejected. Any areas which are unresolved and which require further research should be specified, and how they might be best investigated may also be stated. Good reviews therefore provide a critical evaluation of the published literature as well as important conclusions based on published and reliable evidence. A short, clear and succinct summary should be provided at the end of an invited review, particularly for a long review. The reader should have a clear idea of what is known about a particular topic and what is yet to be known (Box 20.3). Some journals include a box listing 3 to 7 take-home points that link back to the original questions that the invited review sets out to answer. For an invited review, a large number of relevant references are expected, typically numbering 50 to 75. These must be provided in the style of the journal. While a comprehensive list of references are required, those provided should be what the expert author judges to be the most important and pertinent to the topic. Including older references is recommended, particularly those that pre-date the era of electronic search programs, to give acknowledgment to pioneering work so that others do not "re-invent the wheel". Older articles are often better written than those produced more recently and may serve to put certain topics into historical perspective. As many researchers will use invited reviews as a starting point for literature review for their research, care should be taken to ensure that all references are accurately cited, particularly for online journals to ensure correct linking of referenced articles. Only those references that are easily accessible and retrievable should be used. Whether or not to include figures and tables, and the number allowed, depends on individual journal policy and the topic reviewed by the author. Typically, up to ten figures (or 24 figure parts) and up to four tables may be included.

Box 20.3: Common problems with invited reviews

- Poor organization of contents / irrelevant subheadings
- Inclusion of the author's personal views
- Lack of critical evaluation of the available literature
- Problems or unresolved areas not highlighted
- Insufficient references
- Inaccurately quoted references
- No clear take-home message

SUMMARY

An invited review should ideally be topical, current, balanced, accurate, quotable and easily understood, with clear take-home messages (Box. 20.4).

Box 20.4: Take-home points

1. An invited review provides a comprehensive and detailed analysis of recent developments in a specific topic.
2. Important points from a thorough literature review without introduction of new information, a balanced discussion, and an accurate citing of relevant references, are expected.
3. The article should be easily understood with clear take-home messages.

REFERENCES

1. Peh WCG, Ng KH. Basic structure and types of scientific papers. Singapore Med J 2008;49:522-5.
2. Peh WCG, Ng KH. Title and title page. Singapore Med J 2008;49:607-9.
3. Peh WCG, Ng KH. Preparing the references. Singapore Med J 2009;50:659-62.

21 How to Write a Case Report?

Fatema Jawad

WHAT IS A CASE REPORT?

It is reporting a new experience with a patient having an unusual presentation, or laboratory test results different from the recommended and accepted values, rare imaging pictures, or not responding to the standard therapies. The physician is placed in a dilemma as such a case may not be frequently encountered. There can be confusion in the diagnosis or the response to therapy may be slow and the progress unsatisfactory, making it a rare experience and a cause for reporting it for the benefit of other scientists. There can be adverse drug reactions or allergies not seen in every day practice, which by reporting would provide a high index of suspicion for the clinicians.

Case Reports are important as they convey the uniqueness of the presented patient causing the readers and other clinicians to become alerted. They are a basis for improved care of patients as some rare symptom observed may lead to an accurate diagnosis and more effective treatment.

In the past, case reports have introduced many new disorders to the world of science. Examples are of Burkitts lymphoma, acquired immuno deficiency syndrome and Creutzfeldt-Jakob disease.

Occasionally severe adverse effects of drugs are published, providing an evidence to look out for them as reported by patients and the treatment instituted without loosing time. Unusual histopathology findings in diagnosing a rare disease can be a guideline to readers to remind them of the case. A case report can at times form a basis for further studies, case controlled or cohort, on a larger patient population, to get more accurate results. "Case Reports are the first line of evidence in documenting clinical phenomenon in the peer reviewed literature".

THE FIRST STEP TO BE TAKEN

All the necessary information on the case should be collected on a worksheet. This provides accuracy and no point will be missed out. There should be an informed consent of the patient and the ethical review board of the institution. Photographs or histopathology slide pictures or micrographs should be collected if they have to be included.

WRITING THE CASE

Title

This should be short and informative and convey the contents of the case. Abbreviations are not included in the title. Simplicity is appreciated and fancy titles should be avoided as they cause confusion. The title attracts readership. The title is followed by the names of the authors and their institutions.

Abstract

This should have the full information in an abridged form on the case in approximately 250 words (one must always refer to instructions to authors of a particular journal before preparing an abstract). The abstract should cover the background, the case description and the relevant discussion. It should, however, be written in a paragraph form including all these sections of the case.

It begins with the objective—why is the case being reported. This is followed by the salient features of the case, followed by methods used for care of the patient, outcome of the treatment, what the case contributes to literature and the conclusion. The abstract is the most read part of an article and its accuracy will attract readership.

Key Words

Three to five important terms from the case report are quoted for assisting Literature Search.

Introduction

This section starts with the reason for selecting the particular case and what it would contribute to literature. The rarity of the case should be stated which provides the merits for publication. What is already known on the subject and what has been published must be focused and quoted with the supporting pertinent references. The differences between the two are to be highlighted.

The introduction ought not to be more than three paragraphs and written in the present tense. It should end with "We report a case of this extremely rare presentation.....".

The statement to be avoided is "This is the first reported case in the country."

Case Report

All relevant data on the patient is included in this section in a summary form. The demographic information which includes age, gender, ethnicity, race and where necessary, the occupation, is precisely stated. In some cases diet may have played an important role, especially in nutritional deficiency cases, and this has to be noted in detail.

The mode of presentation, the essential physical examination findings, significant laboratory reports, other diagnostic test results are important aspects of the case report and should be included. To support the results, tables or graphs are used. Histopathology slides, X-rays or CT scans form an integral part of the case report. Occasionally a part of the body is photographed, which is done in a manner to observe anonymity. The precise treatment is stated with the exact doses of the drugs prescribed and route of administration. Any side effects encountered, especially allergic reactions are accurately documented.

If a new technique has been used in the treatment and found successful, it should be highlighted or any procedure undertaken should be briefly described. The findings at the last visit of the patient should be documented to identify the outcome.

Discussion

This is written in a structured format to make it simple and relevant. It should be able to prove the accuracy and validity of the case presented. It begins with the unusual aspects of the case supported by the physical findings, laboratory reports and results of other investigations and any new procedures or innovations used.

The results are compared with other similar published literature to note the difference. The differences are then justified or reasons given according to hypothesis used. What could be the practical applicability of the case has to be emphasized in the discussion. A new mode of treatment, if used, and has provided better results than what is known, needs to be recommended as evidence based.

The discussion ends with a brief summary of the case justifying its importance and what it has added to the existing literature. Recommendations, if valid, are stated for other clinicians.

Conclusion

This is a brief summary of the case focusing on the relevant message derived. It should have justifiable, evidence based facts to help the readers.

Acknowledgment

The contributions of the laboratory, imaging department or colleagues who have helped in reviewing the manuscript or retrieving data should be acknowledged.

References

These should not exceed the numbers permitted by the journal. They are written in Vancouver Style and in ascending order.

SUGGESTED READING

1. Burkitt D, O'Conor GT. Malignant lymphoma in African children. I. A clinical syndrome. Cancer 1961;14:258-69.
2. Gottlieb GJ, Ragaz A, Vogel JV, Friedman-Kien A, Rywlin AM, Weiner EA, Ackerman AB. A preliminary communication on extensively disseminated Kaposi's sarcoma in young homosexual men. Am J Dermatopathol 1981;3: 111-4.
3. Green and Johnson. Writing case reports. J Sports Chiropract and Rehab 2000;14:51-9.
4. Sobieraj DM, Freyer CW. Probable Hypoglycemic Adverse Drug Reaction Associated with Prickly Pear Cactus, Glipizide, and Metformin in a Patient with Type 2 Diabetes Mellitus. The Annals of Pharmacotherapy. Published Online, 1 June 2010, www.theannals.com, DOI 10.1345/aph.1P148.
5. Will RG, Ironside JW, Zeidler M, Cousens SN, Estibeiro K, Alperovitch A, Poser S, Pocchiari M, Hofman A, Smith PG. A new variant of Creutzfeldt-Jakob disease in the UK. Lancet 1996;347:921-5.

22 How to Write a Letter to the Editor

Prakash Mungli

WHAT IS A LETTER TO THE EDITOR?

Letter to editor is the form of communication between the journal audience with the editor, and in doing so with the other readers of the journal. When one reads a published article in a journal and feels something more needs to be added, or when a possible error is discovered, or there is a need to clarify a portion of the text, or to put an alternate and worthy view point, in these a letter will be written to the editor by a reader to share his/her viewpoint.

WHO SHOULD WRITE A LETTER TO THE EDITOR?

All readers of the journal can write his/her views about a published article to make correction of errors, or to add extra information, or to clarify a portion of text published. Letters to the editor, thus, keeps the literature accurate, and authors and editors accountable. Therefore, anyone reading a published article is part of the group who can write a letter to the editor. What is required is that he/she has thoroughly read and thought about the content, be familiar with the other literature published on the topic.

WHY ARE LETTERS IMPORTANT?

Letters to the editor help to maintain and strengthen the evidence of previously published paper on certain area of research. The process is fairly simple: readers provide a critical review in the format of a letter to the editor and have it published. From there, the letter is recorded alongside the original paper in literature indexing systems, thus, helping to clarify the original work and strengthen the evidence.

WHAT SHOULD BE WRITTEN IN LETTER TO EDITOR?

Letters to the editors address the contents of an original journal article for one or more of the following: 1. Identify errors and make a correction; 2. Provide an alternate theory; 3. Provide additional information; 4. Offer additional evidence; 5. Provide a counterpoint.

HOW TO WRITE A LETTER TO THE EDITOR?

Letter to the editor should be carefully constructed keeping the points simple and focused. There should not be any personal comments about the authors, indicating personal or professional anger and dislike. Comments that are included should be backed up with references. Traditional reference formatting should be used in letters the same way they are used in full length articles for the same journal. Letters to editors must be brief yet including the points to be conveyed. Lengthy details on original article need not be written, the letter needs to be brief and to the point by staying focused on the primary purpose of writing.

SUGGESTED READING

1. Morgan PP. How to write a letter to the editor that the editor will want to publish. Can Med Assoc J 1985;132(12):1344.
2. Johnson C, Green B. How to write a letter to the editor: an author's guide. J Chiropr Med 2006;5(4):144-7.

Section 5
Miscellaneous

23 Managing Scientific Literature: Editor's Note

Vidya KM, Ranganathan K

INTRODUCTION

Scientific writing and publishing has become an essential part of medical sciences. Undergraduates, postgraduates and senior faculty members in the different specialties have now become aware of the importance of recording as well as publishing their case reports, original studies and reviews. In this context, it is imperative that the author not only follows the *'instruction to the authors'* of the particular journal he/she is submitting to, but should also know the inner workings of the editorial committee. The editorial committee decides at the first step whether to consider the particular submission for publication and it is responsible for the various processes that the submitted manuscript undergoes which thereby affects the turnaround time of acceptance and publication of the article.

Editor's role in scientific literature is complex and varied. The editor makes critical decisions regarding publication of papers, ranks areas of priority for publication, selects reviewers, moderates the reviewer's comments, answers specific questions from authors and takes final decision about the publication.

The editor also has the additional responsibility of building and maintaining the journal's reputation which he/she most often based on the circulation rates, advertisements placed, negative and positive feedback from readers, number of papers submitted etc.

On the basis of above mentioned functions, the journal selects editors who have performed a certain number of review each year to establish commitment before they can become involved in editorial process, others select editors on the basis of their reputation, and still others select based on the academic excellence and achievements in their concerned field.

This chapter aims at shedding light on the editor's diverse functions and also gives hints to what an editor expects from the scientific manuscripts.

DEALING WITH SUBMISSIONS

Journal Peer Review Systems

- Single editor, external review
- Editorial board with occasional review
- In-house staff and external review
- Additional review

Single Editor, External Review

This review involves a single editor and a pool of reviewers. The editor scans all the submissions, selects only those suitable for the journal and sends each article to more than two reviewers. The editor expects a detailed review which should include suggestions for improving the submission like scientific rigor, study design, data adequacy, and originality of the result, validity of the conclusions, completeness of the cited literature and clarity of writing. If the panel of reviewers disagrees, the submission is sent to a different reviewer. The decision to accept or reject finally rests on the editor.

Speed of decision: It usually takes weeks to months to take decision regarding the submission.

Editorial Board with Occasional Review

Some specialty journals have an editorial board to review all submissions. This board has a range of experts in almost all fields pertaining to the journal. Very rarely external reviewers are used. The chief editor scans the submission and then sends it to the relevant member of the board.

Speed of decision: This review is usually slow as the board members are always in the process of reviewing a large number of submissions. The editor also expects to receive a less detailed review.

In-house Staff and External Review

Most of the scientific journals are peer-reviewed. A peer-reviewed journal is controlled by editorial staff that sends the submitted manuscript to external reviewers. It is a two step process; wherein the manuscript is first reviewed by the editorial team which decides whether the submitted manuscript is within the scope of the journal and, if so, whether it is of an adequate standard to be sent out to external reviewers, secondly, if the paper satisfies the criteria laid down by the editorial board, it is sent to external reviewer.

The in-house staffs review all submissions and are responsible for rejecting 30 to 50% of submissions without external review. In this kind of a review the editorial board is expected to have a good understanding of research methodology, the journals' aims and the readers' interest.

The list below gives the criteria on the basis of which the in-house staff decides whether to send the manuscript for external review or not:

1. The manuscript should fit within the scope of the journal.
2. The manuscript should have followed the 'Instruction to the authors' very strictly.
   a. The manuscript should be accompanied by a covering letter addressed to the editor.
   b. The manuscript should be submitted with a title page containing the main title, running title (with few key words), all the contributing author's full names and their affiliations ,word count of the abstract, word count of the main manuscript and any other details that the particular journal demands. The editorial team includes these under the title: Technical modifications.

Speed of decision: If the article is rejected, the decision is rapid, but if the in-house team feels that the submission is publishable then it sends it to external review and the turnaround time for this may take months.

Additional Review

A submission is sent to additional review when the reviewers disagree and the submission is highly technical. A submission is sent for statistical review after the content has been reviewed by experts.

Speed of decision: Usually decision is delayed.

DEALING WITH REVIEWERS

Selection of Reviewers

Reviewers can be selected by various methods as listed below.

1. The editor usually inherits a database of reviewers listing their field of expertise.
2. Potential reviewers can be selected from the authors who submit their work.
3. Electronic databases like Medline can be searched.

4. Editor can request the author to submit a list, nominating reviewers.

Most often the submissions go for masked reviews to minimize personal bias. The author's identity is removed before submitting the article to the reviewer. The reviewer's identity is also not revealed to the author.

After the reviewer sends in the queries and comments, the responsibility rests on the editor to modify the comments and fine tune them and forward them to the author. The editor usually requests for a detailed reply addressing each query raised by the reviewer which the editor forwards to the author. If the replies from the author are adequate then the reviewer recommends publication, even after this the final decision to publish the particular manuscript rests with the editor.

DEALING WITH AUTHORS

After receiving the comments from the reviewers, the editor/editorial committee decides along one of the following lines: acceptable for publication, acceptable for publication with minor revisions, acceptable only after major revision. If the editor replies as "reconsidered after major revisions" it means that there are high chances that the manuscript is unacceptable for publication.

These letters to corresponding authors are always accompanied by list of detailed queries from the reviewers regarding the manuscript. The editor modifies the main comments from the reviewers and forwards it to the author.

Revisions: The editor sends a communication to the author with the reviewer's comments and requests the author to comply within a stipulated time so that the article is accepted and published.

Letters of rejection are usually sent very quickly when compared to acceptance because most of the PUBMED indexed journals screen and reject the manuscript even before sending it to external review, the purpose being that the editor will not be willing to send poor quality manuscript to the external reviewers. Rejection letters are usually polite and state clearly the reason for rejection which applies both to the initial rejection by the editorial team and the rejection from the external reviewers.

Plagiarism: The editorial board in the initial screening in specialty journals almost always checks for the originality for the submitted manuscript. This is done by a thorough internet (Medline, PUBMED) search on the specific topic. Sometimes, the editorial team communicates with the stalwarts in the particular topic, clarifies the validity of the same and then proceeds with the external review.

Publishing similar papers in two or more journals duplicate or multiple publications is also unacceptable. Most journals ask the authors to give in writing whether the article has been concurrently submitted in another journal or not in a specific copyright form.

Publication Charges

Most of the indexed journals charge for printing color photographs, color graphs and reprints. The details regarding the remittance of the specified amount is usually given in the instructions to the authors. Sometimes, some journals print the first three pages free of charge however, a specific amount for the subsequent pages.

DEALING WITH PRINTERS AND PUBLISHERS

The editor communicates with the publishers regarding the copyediting or technical editing of the manuscript. The copy editor may take about ten to thirty days to process the technical part and communicates with the author directly or via the editor. Copyediting of the manuscript mainly involves English language corrections. The authors incorporate the changes suggested within a short time and then the manuscript becomes a portable document format (pdf) proof. This is the ultimate version immediately before the final print and the editor specifically requests the author not to make anymore changes in the manuscript. The editor also decides the time at which the online version of the journal issue is going to be released and communicates the same to the publishers.

SUGGESTED READING

1. Wagner E, Godlee F, Jefferson T. How to survive peer review. London, BMJ Book, British Medical Journal Publishing Group, 2002.
2. Peat J, Elliot E, Baur L, Keena V. Scientific Writing, Easy when you know how. London, BMJ Book, British Medical Journal Publishing Group, 2002.
3. Hornby AS, Parnwell EC. An English-Reader's Dictionary. 2nd edn, London, Oxford University Press; 1975.
4. O'Connor M: Write successfully in Science. London and New York, E & FN Spon Publication, 1996.
5. Cicutto L:Plagiarism: Avoiding the Peril in Scientific Writing. Chest 2008; 133;579-81.

24 How to Deal with Editors

Amar A Sholapurkar

INTRODUCTION

Once you submit your manuscript to a journal, most of the journals acknowledge receipt of the paper. If you do not receive this within 2 to 3 weeks, it is worth checking by writing a letter to the editor to request for an acknowledgment. The referring process can take time and hence it is better to avoid enquiring about the status of your manuscript for at least 6 to 8 weeks.

Once the manuscript is submitted to a journal, the editor initially evaluates for its appropriateness'. He/she sends the copies to two or three reviewers. These reviewers send back the written comments and suggestions within stipulated time. The editor evaluates to make the decision of the manuscript. The editor will then send you a letter describing the decision as well as the comments by the reviewers.

EDITORIAL DECISION

Journals usually vary in their editorial decisions however most of them will have one of the three decisions, i.e. (1) acceptance without revision, (2) rejection, and (3) revision requested.

Acceptance without Revision/Outright Acceptance

It is unusual for a manuscript to be accepted without revision. Outright acceptance may be a dream for the author however, it is rare especially in top journals. For few journals, acceptance without revision is routine. The high standards of these journals are maintained by the fact of the caliber of the authors who are permitted to publish in them, who are the members of the academy. If you are lucky enough to get your paper accepted without revisions, then you need not have to take any further action until you receive the proofs, however one can write a note thanking the editor.

The editor's decision—Sometimes, the editor's decision is easy. If both the reviewers advice acceptance of the manuscript with no or little revision, then the editor has no problem. On the other hand if both the reviewers reject the manuscript then the decision is still easier where the editor evaluates the comments and rejects the article. Unfortunately, there are instances where the opinion/views of the two reviewers are contradictory. In such case, the editor evaluates the comments of both the reviewers and gives weightage to the best comments. In this case, the editor must be reasonably expert in the subject concerned with the manuscript. Or else the editor will send the manuscript to a third (additional) reviewer to determine the result. The later approach is however time consuming. It is true that editorial board members and reviewers can only suggest, recommend, comment on the manuscript but the final decision must be of the editor.

Outright Rejection

If your manuscript is rejected, this means that the paper doesn't fit into or is inappropriate for that journal. There may be several reasons for rejection of your paper. To the best of my knowledge top journals will have an acceptance rate of only 20 to 30%. Most of the editors will usually use descent words when rejecting the article. They usually use the word "unacceptable" rather than "reject". The editor's letter will give you a clue whether the article is worth submitting to another journal. Sometimes the editor himself/herself will suggest you to submit the article to some journal.

Rejection is very common and hence do not be discouraged or lose your hope to publish further. I still remember, my first manuscript got rejected in 6 journals and still I didn't loose my hope. I kept trying and finally it was accepted in a good journal after making a lot of corrections. Many a times, the editor himself will go through the gist of article [the title, and abstract] and will determine whether it is acceptable or not. He/she will send you a letter of rejection immediately (probably within 2 to 3 days of submission) without sending it to the reviewers. At this instance you are lucky enough as the editor has saved your 2 to 3 months of waiting period. Do not again lose your hopes. The reason why the editor does not prefer to send it to the reviewers is that he/she thinks that the reviewers may also feel the same way and reject.

In case, the editor has sent the paper to the reviewers and then the reviewers reject then you need not have to worry. You will, still have chances of improvement by correcting the manuscript based on the comments of reviewers. The editor usually encloses detailed reasons for rejection provided by the reviewers. The following are the most common reasons for rejection of a paper. The reviewers might have found that:

1. The paper is out of scope of the journal.
2. There are fundamental flaws in the paper.
3. There was nothing significant in your paper which may add to the literature.
4. Your study was a repetition of previous study with no additional findings.
5. You have conducted some improper/wrong/irrelevant statistical tests
6. There was no improvement with respect to previous submissions of the same paper.
7. The paper lacked clarity in writing, readability, organization, and overall quality of the paper.
8. The paper had inappropriate title and abstract, ill-designed figures and tables.
9. Methods were carried out improperly and the results were not up to the mark.
10. The paper had no sound discussion and conclusion.
11. The overall length of article was too much or too small.
12. The authors have not followed the guidelines properly.
13. The paper was not well structured.

Once you receive the letter of rejection (In other words the editor means to say that "We don't like this article" OR "the journal is very pressed for space'), read the letter carefully. If the editor says that the paper doesn't fit into the scope of the journal, then it is best to send it to another journal. Secondly, if the article is rejected because it is too long, and needs major changes, then you can shorten the article and modify the changes according to the reviewer's comments and send it to another journal. Thirdly, if your paper is rejected as a result of defect in the experimental work (Lack of control experiment) then you should consider the necessary repairs according to the comments of the reviewers and resubmit it to the same journal by requesting the editor. If you can make the addition of the control experiment as requested by the reviewers and resubmit it then there are high chances of acceptance. Finally, the most important point to be remembered is that editors are mediators between you and the reviewers. You should not be afraid to talk to the editors as they are good people (with rare exceptions). Remember that they are usually not on the other side [They are on your side] and their only goal is to publish good articles. If your paper is rejected and you honestly think (after careful consideration) that the reviewers have made a superficial or wrong comment/judgment then you can deal with the editor respectfully by defending your work scientifically. At this instance most of the rejected papers may even stand out to be among the published ones but you need to deal with the editors in a cleaver way. In this case, write a letter to the editor in a polite fashion explaining why you think that the decision needs to be reconsidered, but also do not spend much time trying to prove the editor or reviewer wrong. Stress that you are willing to do everything and more to alleviate the reviewers concerns and to improve the paper.

What doesn't help?

- Inflammatory language
- Calling the editors or reviewers
- Bribes or threats
- Blanket statements that the reviewers are unfair
- Statements about your reputation and where you have previously published.

Revision Requested

If you are asked to resubmit your paper after revisions then it is an indication that you are doing well and there are high chances that your paper may be acceptable for publication. Congratulations and cheer up. The letter you may receive, may request for specific changes. If the editor writes to you saying that your paper will be accepted / or is being provisionally acceptable if you make the necessary changes then read the comments carefully. First determine whether the revisions are major or minor.

Most likely you will receive a covering letter from the editor with two or three list of labeled reviewer comments. The covering letter may be something like this–Refer Box 24.1

Box 24.1: Covering Letter from the editor

Dear Author,

The peer review process for your manuscript titled "XYZ" is now complete. It has been determined that your manuscript may be acceptable for publication pending some requested revisions. Please be sure to share this information with all co-authors. Please review the peer review comments and requests carefully and edit the manuscript to respond to them. To expedite the re-review process, please attach to your revised manuscript a point-by-point cover letter detailing the changes you have made in response to the editor or reviewer comments. We sincerely hope that you will undertake the necessary revisions as we believe your manuscript stands to make a valuable contribution to our journal. Please make every effort to address the remaining concerns and to resubmit

---

Contd...

Contd...

your manuscript within one month. If you anticipate an additional delay or do not plan to resubmit your manuscript please notify us as soon as possible. Also, please provide complete and up-to-date contact information for all authors, including titles, credentials, mail addresses, phone numbers and e-mail addresses. Please be sure that you have submitted (uploaded) brief biosketches, email addresses and photographs (as JPEGS, TIFFs or PSDs) for each co-author to be included in the publication. In the meantime, please keep your coauthors appraised of the status of the article. Please click the link below to submit your revised manuscript with cover letter:

.... link...

If you have any questions regarding this process, please feel free to contact the managing editor at: xyz@abcmail.com. If I can answer any questions or you wish to discuss any aspect of the review of your manuscript, please do not hesitate to contact me directly. Thank you once again for submitting your manuscript to our journal. Sincerely,

Editor

At this instance, don't be over confident that your paper will be accepted. Be patience and proceed further. On the other hand you should be happy that you have received a provisionally accepted letter rather than a rejection letter. Now, read the comments carefully and decide if you can make the corrections. If the requested corrections are relatively few, then you should go ahead and make them. In case you have been requested a major revision, you need to step back a step and take a total look at your manuscript and your present status and position. Take care to deal with every comment and correct everything you agree with.

This is a proper way to present a point-by-point response. Refer - Box 24.2 [*Source - Ushma S. Neill, How to write a scientific masterpiece. The JCL Inv 2007 Dec;17(12) 3601*].

Box 24.2: Proper way to present a point-by-point response

Referee Point 1 → The authors make the point that A shows B through C in D cells, but they do not provide any evidence to show that B works through C in an in vivo model of E syndrome or in clinical samples from patients with E syndrome. Demonstrating B functions through C in the F model of E syndrome would be required at a minimum.

Response → We thank this reviewer for his/her critical and helpful evaluation of our manuscript. In response to the reviewer's critique, our manuscript has undergone a major revision. In figure 4 we have added new data in the F model of E syndrome that demonstrate that B goes through C. In figure 5 we investigated B expression in a case series of biopsies from patients with E syndrome to confirm the result in human samples.

Once you have made a covering letter with point by point response, modify or rewrite sentences or sections as necessary in the main manuscript file. Enclose the original manuscript as well as the retyped copies. It is also important to meet the editor's deadline. If you fail to meet the deadline, your revised manuscript may be treated as a new manuscript and again subjected to full review, possibly to different set of reviewers. Once you have made the corrections and resubmit the manuscript in the stipulated time, the editor will go through all the corrections and will reply back within few days. If the corrections are done well and the manuscript is worth publishing in the journal, then the editor is happy to reply back to you with an acceptance letter which will be as follows—Refer Box 24.3.

Box 24.3: Acceptance letter from the editor

Dear Author

I am delighted to inform you that your manuscript titled "XYZ" has been accepted for publication no later than the "abc" issue of the Journal. Please be sure to share this information with all coauthors. At this time we need for you to complete the attached publication agreement and return it as soon as possible. We will be in contact with you during the processing of your manuscript. Please feel free to contact me if you have any questions. I would also ask that you place my e-mail address on your "safe senders list" if you use spam software in your e-mail system. This will avoid unnecessary communication problems during the publication of your manuscript. Thank you for submitting your manuscript to our journal and we hope you will submit other manuscripts for consideration in the future.

Sincerely,
Editor

THE ENTIRE PROCESS OF PUBLISHING A PAPER IN A JOURNAL—REFER THE FIGURE 24.1

The process of publishing scientific literature has been very much simplified .Gone are the days when write ups were sent via conventional post. The internet with virtual reality is in and all the journals have websites into which the article write up can be uploaded. The journal online sites have facilitated fast track submission and decision.

Once the article is submitted, the editorial team screens it and quickly decides whether the article is fit for further processing and if yes, sends it to peer-reviewers immediately. If the submission is found to be out of the scope of the journal, it is rejected. The reviewers also have to respond within a specific time limit, usually two weeks. The reviewer's suggestion is considered and if favorable, the communication for revision is immediately sent to the authors (via email).If the reviewer's opine negatively, then the final decision to reject the article is again rapidly taken by the editor and communicated to the author(s), citing the reasons.

The journal also sets time limit for response from the authors. Editorial team checks the revised submission and decides whether the revised submission will be sent for re-review. After this, the editorial team sends the manuscript for technical editing including language correction and the final manuscript or the proof copy (PDF file format) is sent to the author. No further changes are encouraged.

To conclude, easy online submission, quick editorial review, peer review and rapid time dependent decision has reduced the turn-around time in scientific literature publication.

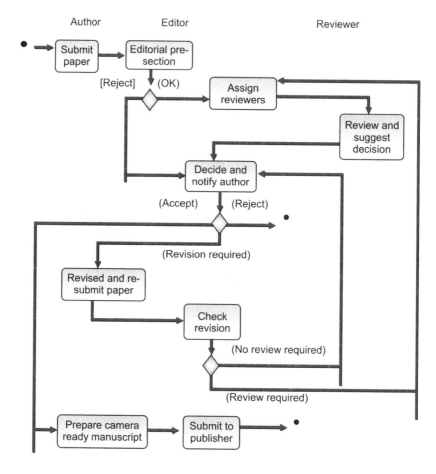

Figure 24.1: The process of publishing a paper in a journal
(Adapted from Micheal Derntl. Basics of research paper writing and publishing (unpublished manuscript – Revision 2.1 September 2009) p. 12)

SUGGESTED READING

1. F Peter Woodford. Scientific writing for graduate students. A manual on the teaching of scientific writing. 1st edn, New York: Rokefeller University press; 1968.
2. Maeve O' Connor, F Peter Woodford. Responding to Editor. In: Maeve O' Connor, F Peter Woodford (Eds). Writing Scientific Papers in English. An ELSE-Ciba Foundation Guide for Authors. 1st edn. England: Pitman Medical Publishing Co Ltd; 1977. pp 70-2.

3. Robert A Day. The Review Process(How to deal with Editors). In:Robert A Day(ed) How to write and publish a scientific paper. 4th edn. New York: Cambridge University Press; 1995. pp. 98-110.

4. Robert Barrass. Scientists must Write. A guide to better writing for scientists, engineers and students. 1st edn. London: Chapman and Hall, 1978.

5. Shakiba B, Salmasian H, Yousefi-Nooraie R, Rohanizadegan M. Factors influencing editors' decision on acceptance or rejection of manuscripts: the authors' perspective. Arch Iran Med 2008;11(3):257-62.

25 Ethical Considerations in Good Publication Practice

Prakash Mungli

INTRODUCTION

Medicine is learnt by experience and experiments. Since centuries, experiments in medicine has been carried about to understand the pathophysiology and treatment of various disorders. Every individual is different due to variation in genetic composition, hence they respond differently with other individuals for the same disease or treatment. This has brought into a new field of research called "pharmacogenomics" or in simple words, individualized medicine. Years of research in medicine have resulted into rapid diagnosis and treatment of various disorders, and continued research is shedding light on unresolved questions. The main goal of medical research is to understand the basic pathophysiology of the disease, methods to diagnose the disease, design a drug to treat the disorder, measure the effectiveness of treatment, and to monitor the treatment and disease progression. Although, great progress has been witnessed in medical research in recent times but nevertheless, there are still many unanswered questions about the functioning of the human body, the causes of diseases (both familiar and novel ones) and the best ways to prevent or cure them. To resolve these issues and to unveil the mystery behind many unresolved questions, medical research is the only means.

ETHICS AND MEDICAL RESEARCH*

Before ethical requirements for medical research were made, physicians in Nazi Germany conducted experiments on prisoners of World War II without their consent, clearly violating the fundaments human rights. Probing into the way the medical research conducted on prisoners of

---

* **Source:** *John R Williams. Ethics and Medical research. In: John R Williams (Ethics unit of world medical association). Medical ethics Manual. 2nd edn. France: World Medical Association 2009; pp 95-111.*

war by a special tribunal at Nuremberg, Germany, some of these physicians were convicted. The judgment by this special tribunal, known as the Nuremberg Code, has served as one of the foundational documents of modern research ethics. The World Medical Association (WMA) was established in 1947, the same year that the Nuremberg Code was set forth. The WMA has taken measures to make sure that all the physicians involved in medical research at least be aware of their ethical obligations. In 1954, the WMA adopted a set of principles for those in research and experimentation. This document was revised and eventually adopted as the Declaration of Helsinki (DOH) in 1964. DOH has been read and revised to include and exclude the certain principles according to the time and needs.

Ethics Review Committee Approval

DOH states that every individual who would like to conduct research on human subjects has to approach ethics committee for approval. All institution who would like to conduct human research has to make institutional ethics committee which includes the legal expert to review the research proposals submitted. In order to obtain approval, researchers must explain the purpose and methodology of the project; demonstrate how research subjects will be recruited, how their consent will be obtained, how their privacy will be protected; specify how the project is being funded; and disclose any potential conflicts of interest on the part of the researchers. The ethics committee must do unbiased evaluation of the research proposal and may accept the study as presented, or ask for changes before it can start, or refuse the approval altogether. Ethics committee has power to monitor the research underway to make sure that the study the researchers fulfill their obligations and they can if necessary stop a project because of serious unexpected adverse events.

Scientific Merit

DOH states that the ethics committee must make sure that the medical research involving human subjects must be justifiable on scientific grounds. This requirement is meant to avoid or eliminate the projects that unlikely to be succeeded due to inadequacy in methods applied for conducting research or which may likely produce trivial results for the amount of risk taken by the subjects under study. Even though, the proposed study may not involve any risk to subjects under study, but still ethics committee must look for the important scientific outcome from the study. All research on animals must conform to ethical guidelines that minimize the number of animals used and prevent unnecessary pain.

Social Value

At the broad outlook, DOH states that ethics committee should make sure that the research must contribute knowledge both to science and the well-being of society in general. The proposed project's objective must address the outcome and outweigh the risks and burdens to research subjects. Furthermore, the populations in which the research is carried out should benefit from the results of the research. Researchers and ethics review committees must ensure that patients are not subjected to tests that unlikely serve any useful social purpose. To approve research proposals and to conduct research which does not contribute significantly to science and society, would mean that it is waste of valuable health resources and such research proposals will weaken the reputation of medical research as a major contributing factor to human health and well-being.

Risks and Benefits

DOH states that ethics committee must look into the risk/benefits aspect of the proposed study once its scientific merit and social worthiness is accepted. It is necessary for the researcher to demonstrate that the risks to the research subjects are not unreasonable or disproportionate to the expected benefits of the research. DOH requires ethics committee to assess the researchers whether they have adequately assessed the risks involved in the study and be sure that they can be managed. If the risk is entirely unknown, then, the ethics committee should not allow the researcher to proceed with the project until some reliable data are available, for example, from laboratory studies or experiments on animals.

Informed Consent

Even the first principle of the Nuremberg Code clearly states that "The voluntary consent of the human subject is absolutely essential", DOH and other research ethics documents recommends that the research subject should have sufficient knowledge and comprehension of the elements of the subject matter involved as to enable him/her to make an understanding and enlightened decision. It also mandates that researchers must obtain informed consent by having the research subject sign a 'consent form' after explaining the study plan and risk involved. Many ethics review committees require the researcher to provide them with the consent form they intend to use for their project. Moreover, research subjects should be informed that they are free to withdraw their consent to participate at any time, even after the project has begun, without any sort of reprisal from the researchers/other physicians and without any compromise of their healthcare.

Confidentiality

All humans are entitled to have their privacy and also apply the same to research subjects with regard to their personal health information. Medical research requires the disclosure of personal health information to others, including the wider scientific community and sometimes the general public. In order to protect privacy, researchers must ensure that they obtain the informed consent of research subjects to use their personal health information for research purposes, which requires that the subjects are told in advance about the uses to which their information is going to be put. As a general rule, the information should be de-identified and should be stored and transmitted securely.

GUIDELINES ON GOOD PUBLICATION PRACTICE*

Study Design and Ethical Approval

Definition

Good research should be well justified, well planned, appropriately designed, and ethically approved. To conduct research at a lower standard may constitute misconduct.

Data Analysis

Definition

Data should be appropriately analyzed but inappropriate analysis does not necessarily amount to misconduct. Fabrication and falsification of data do constitute misconduct.

Authorship

Definition

There are no universally agreed guidelines on the number and sequence of authorship. As a minimum requirement, all the authors must have

---

*Source: The COPE Report 1999. Guidelines on good publication practice. Family Practice 2000;17:218-21

taken part in the study, or contributed to the study, in one or the other way. The award of authorship should balance intellectual contributions to the conception, design, analysis and writing of the study against the collection of data and other routine work. If there is no task that can reasonably be attributed to a particular individual, then that individual should not be credited with authorship. To avoid conflict and confusion about the authorship at the time of manuscript preparation, it is wise to decide on the role of each individuals participating in the study. Accordingly each individual can be credited as authors or as contributors. All those who support the study by means of infrastructure or head of the institutions/departments who support the study indirectly by means of providing moral or financial support must be acknowledged. All authors must take public responsibility for the content of their paper; it can be divided among the authors as individual contribution to the study at the time of manuscript submission.

Conflicts of Interest

Definition

Conflicts of interest implies that the outcome of the study under consideration/publication has biased/modified/not the actual facts, and it may give suspicion on the judgment of author, reviewers, and editors. They have been described as those which, when revealed later, would make a reasonable reader feel misled or deceived. They may be personal, commercial, political, academic or financial. "Financial" interests may include employment, research funding, stock or shared ownership, payment for lectures or travel, consultancies and company support for staff. Such interests, where relevant, must be declared to editors. Editors should also disclose relevant conflicts of interest to their readers.

Peer Review

Definition

Peer reviewers are external experts chosen by editors to provide written opinions, with the aim of improving the study. Choosing the reviewers to review the study submitted to the journal vary from journal to journal. Some editors decide about the reviewer (who will be the one who is known in the specific field of research and would have many publications in such field) to review a study submitted to the journal. Editors usually will send a request mail to selected reviewers about their willingness to review the manuscript and maintain the confidentiality about the manuscript under review. Some editors or journal will ask the authors to suggest three to four reviewers to review their manuscript and also ask authors to mention the names of the reviewers to whom the submitted manuscript is not to be sent for review. Even if authors suggest reviewers to review their submitted manuscript, the final decision about selecting the reviewers will be with editor of the journal.

The duty of confidentiality in the assessment of a manuscript must be maintained by expert reviewers, and this extends to reviewers' colleagues who may be asked (with the editor's permission) to give opinions on specific sections. The submitted manuscript should not be retained or copied. Reviewers and editors should not make any use of the data, arguments, or interpretations, unless they have the authors' permission. Reviewers should provide speedy, accurate, courteous, unbiased and justifiable reports. If reviewers suspect misconduct, they should write in confidence to the editor. Journals should publish accurate descriptions of their peer review selection and appeals processes.

Redundant Publications

Definition

Redundant publication occurs when two or more papers, without full cross reference share the same hypothesis, data, discussion points, or conclusions. Previous publication of an abstract during the proceedings of meetings or during conference or workshop does not prevent from subsequent submission for publication, but full disclosure should be made at the time of submission. Re-publication of a paper in another language is acceptable, provided that there is full and prominent disclosure of its original source at the time of submission. At the time of submission, authors should disclose details of related papers, even if in a different language, and similar papers in press.

Plagiarisms

Definition

Plagiarism ranges from the unreferenced use of others published and unpublished ideas, including research grant applications to submission under "new" authorship of a complete paper, sometimes in a different language. It may occur at any stage of planning, research, writing, or publication: it applies to print and electronic versions. All sources should be disclosed, and if large amounts of other people's written or illustrative material are to be used, permission must be sought.

CONFLICTS OF INTEREST IN MEDICAL RESEARCH*

Conflict of interest exists when an author (or the author's institution), reviewer or editor have financial or personal relationships (also known as dual commitments, competing interests or competing loyalties) that inappropriately influence (bias) his or her actions. Such relationships vary from negligible to great potential for influencing judgment. The potential for conflict of interest can exist as and when an individual believes that the relationship affects his or her scientific judgment. Among all the types of conflicts of interest, financial relationships are the most easily identifiable conflicts of interest and the most likely to undermine the credibility of the journal, the authors, and of science itself. However, conflicts can occur for other reasons such as personal relationships, academic competition, and intellectual passion. Public trust in the peer-review process and the credibility of published articles depends on how well conflict of interest is handled during writing, peer review, and editorial decision making.

Journals now ask to disclose potential conflicts of interest among the authors and also the reviewers at the time of submission and review of original manuscripts and case reports. Disclosure of such relationships is also important in connection with editorials and review articles because it can be more difficult to detect bias in these types of publications than in original research. Editors may use information disclosed in conflict-of-interest and financial-interest statements as a basis for editorial decisions. They should publish this information if they believe it is important in judging the manuscript.

Potential Conflicts of Interest Related to Individual Authors' Commitments

To prevent ambiguity, all authors at the time of submitting a manuscript are asked to disclose whether potential conflicts do exist or not. Authors need to sign a form about conflict of interest in the manuscript on a conflict-of-interest notification page that follows the title page, providing additional detail if necessary. When authors submit a manuscript,

---

* *Reproduced with permission from*—*International Committee of Medical Journal Editors. Ethical Considerations in the Conduct and Reporting of Research: Conflicts of Interest. Available at: http://www.icmje.org/ethical_4conflicts.html. Accessed: 1st August 2010.*

whether an article or a letter, they are responsible for disclosing all financial and personal relationships that might bias their work. Authors should identify individuals who provide writing or other assistance and disclose the funding source for the same.

Potential Conflicts of Interest Related to Commitments of Editors, Journal Staff, or Reviewers

Selection of reviewers to review a manuscript is finally decided by editor of the journal; however, editor can ask the authors to suggest reviewers. Most of the time, editors will avoid selecting external peer reviewers with obvious potential conflicts of interest—for example, those who work in the same department or institution. Most of the journal will ask authors to provide editors with the names of persons they feel should not be asked to review a manuscript because of potential, usually professional, conflicts of interest.

It is the duty of reviewers to disclose to editors any conflicts of interest that could bias their opinions of the manuscript, and they should withdraw themselves from reviewing specific manuscripts if any potential for bias exists. If the reviewer remains silent on the conflict of interest statement, it means either that conflict exists and the reviewer has failed to disclose them or conflicts do not exist. Hence reviewers are asked to state explicitly whether conflicts do exist or not.

Editor of the journal is the one who make final decision on selecting the manuscript and selecting the manuscript to publish after going through reviewers comments and authors response to reviewers comments. Editors who make final decisions about manuscripts must have no personal, professional, or financial involvement in any of the issues they might judge. Conflict of interest also applies to other members of the editorial staff, if they participate in editorial decisions, must provide editors with a current description of their financial interests (as they might relate to editorial judgments) and rescue themselves from any decisions. According to ethical guidelines, either editor or editorial staff must not use information gained through working with manuscripts for private gain. Editors should publish regular disclosure statements about potential conflicts of interests related to the commitments of journal staff.

Authors and Reviewers

Authors should consult the "information for authors" of the journal to which they have chosen to submit a manuscript to determine whether reviews are anonymous. Authors entrust editors, in submitting their manuscript with the results of their scientific work and creative effort on which their reputation and career may depend. Manuscripts must be reviewed with due respect for authors' confidentiality. Authors' rights may be violated by disclosure of the confidential details during review of their manuscript. Reviewers must not be allowed to make copies of the manuscript for their files and must be prohibited from sharing it with others, except with the editor's permission. Reviewers should return or destroy copies of manuscripts after submitting reviews. Reviewers also have rights to confidentiality, which must be respected by the editor. Reviewer's identity must not be revealed to the author or anyone else without the reviewer's permission. Confidentiality may have to be breached if dishonesty or fraud is alleged but otherwise must be honored.

Editors must make clear to their reviewers that manuscripts sent for review are privileged communications and are the private property of the authors. They should not keep copies of rejected manuscripts nor disclose information about manuscripts (including their receipt, content, status in the reviewing process, criticism by reviewers, or ultimate fate) to anyone other than the authors and reviewers. Reviewers and members of the editorial staff must respect the authors' rights by not publicly discussing the authors' work or appropriating their ideas before the manuscript is published. Reviewer comments should not be published or otherwise publicized without permission of the reviewer, author, and editor. Reviewers also may be notified of the editor's decision to accept or reject a manuscript. When reviewers' comments are published, permission from both the reviewers and authors has to be taken. However, editor can send previous reviewer's comments to other persons reviewing the same manuscript, which helps reviewers, learn from the review process.

WEB RESOURCES ON PUBLICATION AND RESEARCH ETHICS

The following links are to web sites that contain information useful to editors on ethical issues.

The list is divided generally into Research Ethics and Publication Ethics, although the two topics are closely related.

RESEARCH ETHICS

American Association of Medical Colleges (AAMC)*
http://www.aamc.org/research/dbr/compliance/models.htm

Declaration of Helsinki
http://www.wma.net/e/policy/pdf/17c.pdf

Food and Drug Administration (United States)
http://www.fda.gov/oc/gcp/default.htm

Health Care Ethics Committee Forum (HEC Forum)
http://www.kluweronline.com/issn/0956-2737

Indian Council of Medical Research
http://www.icmr.nic.in/ethical.pdf

*National Institutes of Health**
http://www.nih.gov/sigs/bioethics/

Public Responsibility in Medicine & Research (PRIM&R)
http://www.primr.org/

University of Pittsburgh
http://www.edc.gsph.pitt.edu/survival/

United States Federal Regulations
http://www.access.gpo.gov/cgi-bin/cfrassemble.cgi?title=199845

World Medical Association (WMA) - The Declaration of Helsinki, plus basic and ethical principles for medical research.
http://www.wma.net/e/policy/17-c_e.html

PUBLICATION ETHICS

American Chemical Society (ACS)
http://pubs.acs.org/instruct/ethic.html

American Medical Writers Association (AMWA)
http://www.amwa.org/

American Statistical Association
http://www.amstat.org/profession/ethicalstatistics.html

*BioMed Central (BNC) Medical Ethics**
http://www.biomedcentral.com/1472-6939/

*BMJ resources: **
http://bmj.com/cgi/collection

British Healthcare Internet Association (BHIA)
http://www.bhia.org/reference/documents/
recommend_webquality.htm

Centre for Enquiry into Health and Allied Themes (CEHAT)
http://www.cehat.org/initiatives1.html or http://
www.hsph.harvard.edu/bioethics/guidelines/ethical.html

Clinical Research Workshops
http://ethics.ucsd.edu/workshops/CRW/human.htm

Committee on Publication Ethics (COPE) *
http://www.publicationethics.org.uk/

Council of Science Editors, Inc. (CSE)
http://www.councilscienceeditors.org/

Danish Committee on Scientific Dishonesty
http://www.forsk.dk/eng/uvvu/publ/index.htm

European Association of Science Editors (EASE)
http://www.ease.org.uk/

International Committee of Medical Journal Editors (ICMJE), a.k.a. Vancouver Group
http://www.icmje.org

Journal of the American Medical Association (JAMA)*
http://jama.ama-assn.org/info/auinst.html

Journal of Medical Internet Research
http://www.jmir.org/instruction.htm

Lay publication codes of conduct (listed by country and topic)
http://www.presswise.org.uk/display_page.php?id=40

Medical College Of Ohio*
http://www.mco.edu/lib/instr/libinsta.html

National Library of Medicine (NLM)
http://www.nlm.nih.gov/

New England Journal of Medicine
http://www.nejm.org/hfa/policies.asp

Office of Research Integrity (ORI)*
http://ori.dhhs.gov/html/policies/introduction.asp

Online Ethics Center for Engineering and Science at Case Western Reserve University
http://onlineethics.org/reseth/edu.html

Online Science Ethics Resources
http://www.chem.vt.edu/ethics/vinny/ethxonline.html#institutions

Pharmaceutical company good publication practices guidelines
http://www.gpp-guidelines.org/

Poynter Institute
http://poynter.org/

Society for Neuroscience
http://web.sfn.org/content/Publications/Guidelines2/index.html

SUGGESTED READING

1. International Committee of Medical Journal Editors. Ethical Considerations in the Conduct and Reporting of Research: Conflicts of Interest. Available at: http://www.icmje.org/ethical_4conflicts.html. Accessed: 1st August 2010.
2. The *COPE Report 1999. Guidelines on good publication practice.* Family Practice 2000;17:218–21.
3. John R Williams. Ethics and Medical research. In: John R Williams (Ethics unit of world medical association). Medical ethics Manual. 2nd edn. France: World Medical Association; 2009. pp 95-111.

26 Understanding Informed Consent

Sumanth Prasad

INTRODUCTION

India is increasingly popular for clinical research. A statutory legal obligation in India specifies that researchers should explain to the participants the nature, purpose, risks and benefits of a proposed research as well as alternatives to the process. Efforts to protect the subject's rights and safety should be a principal concern in every clinical study. Many patients state during interview that they had taken trial medications because their doctor asked them to, but had no awareness of what the drugs were and their potential effects. Without exception these patients were very poor, and clearly felt their doctors to be superior in status and intelligence.

Much has been written in the medical literature on why informed consent is so important and how does it differ theoretically and in practice. At present, the level of information given to obtain informed consent can vary widely between individuals. But obligation to obtain the patient's consent is based on ethical principles, legal requirements and professional policies

THE MEANING AND NEED FOR INFORMED CONSENT*

Informed consent is the process, dialog and invitation for the fully informed patient to participate in choices about his/her healthcare and is simply memorialized in the signature or mark. It originates from the legal and ethical right of the patient to direct what happens to his/her body and from the ethical duty of the physician to involve the patient in healthcare decisions. Informed consent implies that a discussion has taken place about basic elements of consent.

---

* *Source — Liesegang TJ .The meaning and need for informed consent in research—Indian J Ophthalmol 2007:55(1):1-3.*

What about consent for participation in research?

Research implies a systematic investigation, research development, testing or evaluation that is designed to develop or contribute to generalized knowledge. Research differs from conventional therapy not only in the comparative uncertainty of risks and benefits, but also the difference in objectives. Patients who volunteer for medical research face some risks. The investigator has dual loyalties to both the protocol and to the patient, perhaps in that order. For participation in research, the basic elements and additional elements of informed consent are required to be followed along with the clinical trials volunteer bill of rights.

Does publication of a case report require subject consent?

If, before an intervention is performed, a medical specialist considers publishing the results of a series of cases, then the local ethical review board approval and informed consent are required. In practice, physicians are permitted to use innovative therapeutic techniques or off-label medications, but if they attempt to gain systematic knowledge from the intervention (e.g. by doing multiple cases or from researching multiple records) then informed consent and local ethical review board approval is required.

ETHICAL PRINCIPLES OF INFORMED CONSENT*

In 1979, the Belmont report outlined three fundamental ethical principles for the protection of human subjects in biomedical and social research: (1) Respect for persons (2) Beneficence, and (3) Justice. According to the report, clinical research must "maximize possible benefits and minimize possible harms." These three principles help researchers, clinicians, study participants and Institutional Review Boards (IRBs) to understand the ethical issues inherent in an informed consent process.

1. Respect for Persons

The principle of respect for persons requires that people should be respected regardless of age, race, gender, and socio-economic status. Respect of persons includes two ethical convictions: first, that well informed people have a fundamental right of saying yes or no in medical research; and second, those persons (such as children, the elderly the

---

* *Source*—*The Belmont Report, April 18, 1979 http://www.fda.gov/oc/ohrt/irbs/ belmont.html*

mentally ill, or prisoners) incapable of making any decision without the assistance of a guardian or caregiver, must receive protection.

2. Beneficence

The second principle means that the goal of research is to maximize the benefits of a drug/intervention under investigation while minimizing the risks to study subjects. Clinical trials must secure the well being of all study participants and protect them from any harm, as well as ensure that they experience the possible benefits of involvement. The principle also means that the potential for risks must be justified by the greater good to the society. Balancing the risks and the benefits is thus, an important consideration.

3. Justice

The third principle means that the benefits and risks of research are shared among different strata of society. The principle of justice gives rise to moral requirements that there be fair procedures and outcomes in the selection of research subjects. Justice is relevant to the selection of subjects at two levels: the individual level and the social level. Individual justice in the selection of subjects would require that researchers exhibit fairness—thus, they should not offer potentially beneficial research only to some patients who are in their favor, or select only undesirable persons for risky research. Clinical trial must be cautious on matters of informed consent when they deal with disadvantaged people like the poor, the sick and the institutionalized. Most clinical trials have a disproportionate number of women, poor, illiterate and patients admitted to general wards in their trials. These participants are too weak to ask the related questions (questions that the ICMR guidelines say are every volunteer's right). Too often these participants bear the risk of a study and the rich and powerful receive its benefits.

INFORMED CONSENT MEASURES*

No clinical investigator may involve a human being as a subject in research unless the investigator has obtained the legally effective informed consent from the subject. Informed Consent is a written

---

* *Source—A Guide to Informed Consent   http://www.fda.gov/oc/ohrt/IRBS/ informedconsent.html*

notification to human subjects involved in clinical investigations that provides them with sufficient opportunity to consider whether or not to participate in the study.

An investigator shall seek consent only under circumstances that provide the subject or the representative sufficient opportunity to consider whether or not to participate and that minimize the possibility of coercion or undue influence. The information that is given to the subject or the representative shall be in language which is understandable.

No informed consent, whether oral or written, may include any exculpatory language through which the subject or the representative is made to waive any legal rights, or releases the investigator, the sponsor, the institution, or its agents from liability for negligence.

1. The written consent form must be approved by the Institutional Review Board (IRB) and contain the following basic elements:*

   - A statement that the study involves research, an explanation of the purposes of the research and the expected duration of the subject's participation, a description of the procedures to be followed and identification of any procedures which are experimental
   - A description of any reasonably foreseeable risks or discomforts to the subject
   - A description of any benefits to the subject or to others which may reasonably be expected from the research
   - A disclosure of appropriate alternative procedures or courses of treatment, if any, that might be advantageous to the subject
   - A statement describing the extent, if any, to which confidentiality of records identifying the subject will be maintained and that notes the possibility that the Food and Drug Administration may inspect the records
   - For research involving more than minimal risk, an explanation as to whether any compensation and an explanation as to whether any medical treatments are available if injury occurs and, if so, what they consist of?
   - An explanation of whom to contact for answers to pertinent questions about the research and research subjects' rights, and in the event of a research-related injury to the subject.

---

* *Source — The Belmont Report, April 18, 1979 http://www.fda.gov/oc/ohrt/irbs/ belmont.html*

- A statement that participation is voluntary, that refusal to participate will involve no penalty or loss of benefits to which the subject is otherwise entitled, and that the subject may discontinue participation at any time without penalty or loss of benefits to which the subject is otherwise entitled.

Additional Elements of Informed Consent*

When appropriate, one or more of the following elements of information must be provided to each subject:

- A statement that a particular treatment or procedure may involve risks to the subject (or to the embryo or fetus, if the subject is pregnant) which are currently unforeseeable
- Anticipated circumstances under which the subject's participation may be terminated by the investigator without regard to the subject's consent
- Any additional costs to the subject that may result from participation in the research
- A statement that, significant new findings developed during the course of the research which may relate to the subject's willingness to continue participation will be provided to the subject
- The approximate number of subject's involved in the study.

THE CLINICAL TRIAL VOLUNTEER'S BILL OF RIGHTS**

Any volunteer who gives his or her consent to participate in a clinical trial or who is asked to give his or her consent on behalf of another has the following rights:

- To be told the purpose of the clinical trial
- To be told about all the risks, side effects or discomforts that might be reasonably expected
- To be told of any benefits that can be reasonably expected
- To be told what will happen in the study and whether any procedures, drugs or devices are different than those that are used as standard medical treatment
- To be told about options available and how they may be better or worse than being in a clinical trial

---

* *Source—A Guide to Informed Consent http://www.fda.gov/oc/ohrt/IRBS/ informedconsent.html*

** *Guidelines for writing informed consent documents. www.Ohsr.od.nih.gov/info/ sheet6.html*

- To be allowed to ask any questions about the trial before giving consent and at any time during the course of the study
- To be allowed ample time, without pressure, to decide whether to consent or not to consent to participate
- To refuse to participate, for any reason, before and after the trial has started
- To receive a signed and dated copy of the informed consent form
- To be told of any medical treatments available if complications occur during the trial.

DIFFICULTIES IN OBTAINING INFORMED CONSENT

There are many variables that would affect the level of autonomy.

Ethnicity and cultural beliefs play a critical role in patient recruitment. Many ethnicities do not seek medical help until issues have a risen. Furthermore, the concept of research is unfamiliar to them. Therefore, it is a challenge to convince this population to participate in research. Recruitment of subjects is especially difficult in populations who share the cultural belief that women are considered property of their husband. This adds another problematic dimension since consent is not granted by the patient herself, but from her husband. In such a situation, proper communications plays a key role in explaining written consent.

The *language barriers* also cannot be easily brushed. With innumerable Indian languages spoken in an area and several dialects of the same language, during communication with an edentulous and illiterate elderly individual, an attempt at extensive explanation may easily turn into a misinformed consent.

SITUATIONS WHERE CONSENT MAY NOT BE OBTAINED

1. Medical Emergencies: The well-being of the patient is paramount and medical rather than legal considerations come first.
2. In case of person suffering from a notifiable disease: In case of AIDS/HIV positive patients, the position in India regarding its being a notifiable disease or not is not yet clear. However, in England the Public Health (Infectious Diseases) Regulations, 1988 extend the provisions of notifiable diseases to AIDS but not to persons who are HIV positive.
3. Immigrants.
4. Members of Armed Forces.
5. Handlers of food and dairymen.
6. New admission to prisons.

7. In case of a person where a court may order for psychiatric examination or treatment.

8. Under Section 53 (1) of the Code of Criminal Procedure, a person can be examined at request of the police, by use of force. Section 53 (2) lays down that whenever a female is to be examined, it shall be made only by, or under the supervision of a female doctor.

9. Informed consent may not be obtained for research involving more than minimal risk.

10. In studies where the consent process may adversely impact the findings by disclosing too much information and creating a bias.

When Consent is not Valid

Consent given under fear, fraud or misrepresentation of facts or by a person who is ignorant of the implications of the consent, or who is under 12 years of age is invalid (Sec. 90 I.P.C.). In most of the cases filed against the doctors it is alleged that no consent was obtained. Obtaining of consent will thus, be a cornerstone of protection against litigation.

SUGGESTIONS FOR WRITING INFORMED CONSENT DOCUMENTS *

When an investigator writes or reviews a research consent document, she/he should ask the following questions:

Question 1: Is it written at a reading level understandable to research subjects?

A general rule of thumb is that consent documents should be written so that they are understandable to people who have not graduated from high school. The reading level of a document is more difficult if it contains long sentences, words with more than two syllables, and continuous run-on text. Use nonscientific/nonmedical words and break the text into short sections.

Question 2: Is the document formatted well? Does it have headings which break the text into short sections?

Question 3: Does the document contain the basic elements for informed consent and are they presented in a clear, easy-to-understand way? Even though the printed consent form incorporates some of the elements of consent, depending on the particular research study, it may be useful to include the information a second time but in a simpler form.

---

* *Source*—*Guidelines for writing informed consent documents. www.Ohsr.od.nih.gov/ info/sheet6.html*

Question 4: Can the document be shortened without compromising clarity or other requirements? Usually, before a person agrees to take part in a research study, he/she not only reads a written consent document but also discusses the study with a researcher. A suggestion when writing consent documents is to assume that prospective subjects will not talk to a researcher (or research nurse) at all about the study and that all their information will come entirely from the consent document. If this approach is used the document is more likely to be clear, complete, devoid of medical/scientific terminology and able to "stand alone."

THE USE OF HEADINGS TO FORMAT INFORMED CONSENT DOCUMENTS*

The use of headings in informed consent documents helps to ensure that all the basic elements of informed consent are conveyed to the prospective research subject in a simple and efficient way. Headings promote comprehension and readability. The following headings are included in the Clinical Center consent writing module of Prototype.

1. Introduction: starting with pleasing words such as, "We invite you . . ." and ending with, ". . . personal physician or other health professional."
2. Why is this research being done?
3. Why are you being invited to participate?
4. How many people will take part in this research study?
5. How long will you take part in this research study?
6. What do we do to decide if you are eligible for this research study?
7. What procedures, drugs or other treatments are involved in this research study?
8. What are the risks and discomforts of this research study?
9. Are there any benefits to you if you take part in this research study?
10. What other choices do you have?
11. Are there reasons that your research participation may end early?
12. What will happen when the research study is over?
13. Will your clinical and other test results be shared with you?
14. Will the results of this research study be shared with you?
15. Will any of your blood, tissue or other samples be stored and used for research in the future?
16. Will you receive any compensation (money or other) for taking part in this research study?

Source—A Guide to Informed Consent http://www.fda.gov/oc/ohrt/IRBS/ informedconsent.html

CONCLUSION

Informed consent refers to participants' agreement that they are willing to take part in the research, having been told what they will be expected to do during the research. They must be given enough information about what they will be expected to do during the research procedure that they can reasonably make an informed decision about whether they agree to participate or not, both verbally and in writing in a manner and language that the participants know and understand. The greater the risk to participants, the greater is the need for it. There should be no compulsion to participate, although positive incentives can be offered. Informed consent is essential to protect the participants, not the researchers and institutions.

SUGGESTED READING

1. A Guide to Informed Consent http://www.fda.gov/oc/ohrt/IRBS/informedconsent.html
2. Consumer Protection Act and Medical Profession—Consent http://www.medindia.net/indian_health_act/consumer_protection_act_and_medical_profession_consent.htm
3. Guidelines for writing informed consent documents. www.Ohsr.od.nih.gov/info/sheet6.html
4. Informed consent: Legal theory and clinical practice. By Jessica W. Berg, Paul S. Appelbaum. 2nd edn.
5. Liesegang TJ .The meaning and need for informed consent in research—Indian J Ophthalmol 2007;55(1):1-3.
6. The Belmont Report, April 18, 1979 http://www.fda.gov/oc/ohrt/irbs/belmont.html
7. WMA Declaration of Helsinki—Ethical Principles for Medical Research Involving Human Subjects
8. www.icmr.nic.in/ethical_guidelines.

27 English Language, Abbreviations and Acronyms in Medical Writing

Prakash Mungli

ENGLISH LANGUAGE

Language converts human imagination to reality, making human culture and science possible. English has been the language of the scientific community ever since the research has started to expand. Now scientists all over the world are obliged to use English to communicate their research findings. Since English is not the native language in most part of the world, it clearly affects the communication of science. The way researcher writes in English depends largely on his or familiarity with the language. Most of the time the thought process will be in the native language and researcher has to translate it into English to communicate. During this process, the chances of misinterpretation by both the author and reader may arise. Since scientist is not expected to be either a professional writer or a translator but for the sake of communicating, the scientific community has to compromise on style of presentation, provided they are within the bounds of English grammar.

There is no standard scientific English against which authors can compare a text, so it is difficult to evaluate the style of a scientific publication. Since there is no standard scientific English, hence local peculiarities, word preference and style of presentation by authors from various countries clearly prevail in some journals, depending on the level of copy-editing of the final text by editors and publishers. Such variations in the use of English due to the author's native language and cultural background not only make a text more difficult to understand and distract the reader from the content, but also hold the danger that the meaning and content of a sentence is diluted or misinterpreted by a reader. Thus, editors and publishing house should recognize locally favored words and phrases, and eventually avoided, to increase the clarity of scientific communication. In general, scientific communication recently made easier by the worldwide web, email and electronic journals could contribute to a convergence towards a global consensus for the English language.

The English alphabet of only 26 characters has produced more than a half a million individual words, the most in any language. Scientific and technical English freely use several logographic characters with the alphabetic, e.g. signs for infinity (α), plus (+), percentage (%), equality (=), and many others. Computer language and programming have greatly expanded this inclusion.

ABBREVIATION

Since ages, as the human culture diversified, many new languages evolved and words became more numerous and more complex. Many writers for emperors started using abbreviations for long sentences or commonly used words to limit the time and space, and may be because of laziness, even when space and time was not limited. This habit of using abbreviations for long sentences and commonly used words continued. Subsequent scientific innovation and communication further stretched the vocabulary. English being used as scientific and technical language to communicate, started freely using several logographic characters for commonly used words, e.g. signs for infinity (α), plus (+), percentage (%), equality (=), and many others. Invention of computer language and programming has greatly expanded this inclusion.

The word abbreviation (word simplification) refers to any shortened form of a word or a phrase, some have used initialism or alphabetism to refer to an abbreviation formed simply from and used simply as a string of initials. Abbreviation can take several forms. *Clipping* applies equally to spoken and written words; for example—ad for advertisement. *Titular contraction* applies to the written word and although contracted in print, these titles are automatically expanded or pronounced in their complete forms when read or spoken, for example—Mr, Dr. *Abbreviation by initialism* can be applied to group of words by substituting initial letters for the individual words. This practice goes back to its Latin origin, with , i.e. (id est, that is to say), q.e.d. (quod erat demonstrandum, that was to be proved), and, e.g. (exempli gratia, for example). The most common form of initialism simply replaces the entire word in a phrase with the first letter. Yet another variant takes the initial letters of distinct syllables of the word, such as ECG for electrocardiogram. Some governmental initialism is now intrinsic parts of medical language, such as FDA (Food and Drug Administration of the US Department of Health and Human Services) or NHS (the UK National Health Service). The general public may not recognize most abbreviations, but certainly most laymen understand DNA, RNA, and AIDS because of their repeated usage in written and spoken language. Computer and electronic communication has become a necessity in modern life in all disciplines and hence the use of computer language. Twenty-first century language will change to reflect the demands of society and science. This change will challenge not only the sentence formation but also the rules of punctuation, grammar, and capitalization.

THE RISE OF THE ACRONYM

In 1943, David Davis of Bell Laboratories coined the term acronym as the name for a word created from the first letters of each word in a series of words. Although the term acronym is widely used to describe any abbreviation formed from initial letters, most dictionaries define acronym to mean "a word" in its original sense, while some include a secondary indication of usage, attributing to acronym the same meaning as that of initialism. The condensation of a word or phrase into a pronounceable initialism (acronym) seems to be a fairly recent invention. The line between simple initialism and pronounceable acronym can be indistinct (e.g. ELISA) although general usage favors the case for simple initialism.

Few examples of different types of acronyms and initialism used in scientific and general community are: 1. Pronounced as a word, containing only initial letters; AIDS: Acquired Immune Deficiency Syndrome, Scuba: Self-contained underwater breathing apparatus. 2. Pronounced as a word, containing non-initial letters: Amphetamine: alpha-methyl-phenethylamine, Radar: radio detection and ranging. 3. Pronounced as a word or names of letters, depending on speaker or context; FAQ: Frequently Asked Questions. 4. Pronounced as a combination of names of letters and a word: CD-ROM: Compact Disc read-only memory, JPEG: Joint Photographic Experts Group. 5. Pronounced only as the names of letters; BBC: British Broadcasting Corporation, DNA: deoxyribonucleic acid. 6. Pronounced as the names of letters but with a shortcut; IEEE: Institute of Electrical and Electronics Engineers. 7. Shortcut incorporated into name; W3C: World Wide Web Consortium, E3: Electronic Entertainment Exposition. 8. Multi-layered acronyms; PAC-3: PATRIOT Advanced Capability 3, i.e. Phased Array Tracking RADAR Intercept on Target, i.e. RAdio Detection And Ranging, VHDL: *VHSIC* hardware description language, where VHSIC stands for very-high-speed integrated circuit. 9. Recursive acronyms, in which the abbreviation refers to itself; GNU: *GNU's not Unix*, LAME: *LAME Ain't an MP3* Encoder. 10. Pseudo-acronyms consisting of a sequence of characters which, when pronounced as intended, invoke other longer words with less typing (internet slang); CQ: "Seek you", a code used by radio operators, Q8: "Kuwait". 11. Initialisms whose last abbreviated word is often redundantly included anyway; HIV virus: *Human Immunodeficiency Virus* virus, ATM machine: *Automated Teller Machine* machine.

Acronyms are firmly fixed in speech and writing, providing great value in modern communication. However, there is widespread evidence of overuse in technical writing and it may be wise to follow some simple rules for acronymology:

- An acronym is at least three letters
- The word must be easily pronounceable
- It must simplify communication
- An acronym should have utility beyond a single paper/report
- Spell out the complete term at first usage
- Do not put the reader in the position of having to refer back to a key of novel abbreviations. It is preferable to spell out most repetitive phrases.

SUGGESTED READING

1. Bloom DA. Acronyms, abbreviations and initialisms. BJU Int 2000; 86(1):1-6. Review.
2. Netzel R, Perez-Iratxeta C, Bork P, Andrade MA. The way we write. EMBO Rep 2003;4(5):446-51.

28 Abbreviations for Units of Measurements

KL Bairy

INTRODUCTION

Abbreviations for most units of measurements use small letters and periods. The few exceptions that use capital letters are noted below. Temperature abbreviations use capitals because they come from proper nouns. Measures of mass or weight of types of tons are usually capitalized when abbreviated. Abbreviations for metric units, including temperatures (Kelvin or Celsius), do not end with periods. Temperature abbreviations are used in all types of writing. Other abbreviations of measurements are limited to lists, charts, technical writing, and informal writing. In standard formal English, they are spelled out. If you spell out the number, spell out the unit of measurement.

UNITS OF TIME

The most frequent units of time used in the biological sciences are:

Year	yr
Day	d
Hour	hr
Minute	min
Second	sec or s
Millisecond	msec

UNITS OF pH

In contrast to other units, one should report pH with the unit before the number: e.g. pH 8.2. When reporting a series of pH values, report the unit only at the beginning: e.g. buffered to pH 3, 5, 7, and 9....

UNITS OF CONCENTRATION

Concentration usually refers to a mass/volume relationship.

Percent (%)	= Grams solute/100 ml solvent; To convert to molar concentration multiply grams by 10, then divide by the formula weight (FW) of the solute.
Morality (M)	= Moles solute per liter of solvent For example, 1 M = 1 mole/liter; where, 1 mole = 6.023×10^{23} molecules = 1 molecular weight (MW) ~ 1 formula weight (FW) Molarity may also be expressed as mM (millimolar), where 1 mM equals 10^{-3} M, when working with low concentrations.
Salinity	= Grams total solutes per kg of seawater Salinity is usually expressed as "parts per thousand" = ppt. Coastal seawater has approximately 30-32 g solutes per kg = 30-32 ppt salinity.

UNITS OF TEMPERATURE

Kelvin   = K
Celsius   = C
Fahrenheit = F
   Fahrenheit (F) to Celsius (C) Conversion
   (degrees F - 32) x 5/9 = degrees C
   Celsius (C) to Fahrenheit (F) Conversion
   (degrees C x 9/5) + 32 = degrees F

UNITS OF LIQUID VOLUMES

Microliters	= μl
Milliliters	= ml
Liters	= L
Fluid ounces	= fl oz
Pints	= pt
Quarts	= qt
Teaspoons	= tsp
Tablespoons	= tbsp
Cups	= c
US gallons	= US gal

METRIC EQUIVALENTS

1 L = 1000 ml = 2.113 pt = 1.06 qt = 0.264 US gal
1 ml (or cm^3) = 1000 μl = 0.03 fl oz

Metric Unit	Multiplied by	= English Unit
Milliliters	0.02957	fluid ounces
Liters	2.13	pints
Liters	1.0567	quarts

ENGLISH EQUIVALENTS

1 US gal = 4 qt = 8 pt = 128 fl oz = 3.785 L
1 qt = 2 pt = 32 fl oz = 946.4 ml or 0.9464 L
1 pt = 16 fl oz = 473.2 ml or 0.213 L
1 fl oz = 29.57 ml

English Unit	Multiplied by	= Metric Unit
Teaspoons	5	milliliters
Tablespoons	15	milliliters
Fluid ounces	29.57	milliliters
cups	0.24	liters
pints	0.4732	liters
quarts	0.9464	liters
US gallons	3.785	liters

UNITS OF VOLUME

Metric Equivalents

1 cm^3 (or cc) = 1000 mm^3 = 0.061 in^3
1 m^3 = 10^3 cm^3 = 61,024 in^3 = 35.31 ft^3 = 1.308 yd^3

Metric Unit	Multiplied by	= English Unit
Cubic centimeters (cm^3)	0.061	cubic inches (in^3)
Cubic meters (m^3)	35.31	cubic feet (ft^3)
Cubic meters	1.308	cubic yards (yd^3)

English Equivalents

1 ft^3 = 1,728 in^3 = 28,317 cm^3 = 0.02832 m^3
1 yd^3 = 27 ft^3 = 0.7646 m^3

English Unit	Multiplied by	= Metric Unit
Cubic inches	16.393	cubic centimeters
Cubic feet	0.03	cubic meters
Cubic yards	0.76	cubic meters

UNITS OF MASS

Metric Equivalents
1 mt (metric ton) = 1000 kg = 2,205 lb
1 kg = 1000 g = 2.205 lb = 35.2802 oz
1 g = 1000 mg = 10^6 ng = 10^9 pg

Metric Unit	Multiplied by	= English Unit
Gram (g)	0.035	ounces (oz)
Kilogram (kg)	2.2	pounds (lb)
Metric ton (mt)	1.102	ton (t)

English Equivalents

1 ton = 2000 lb = 907.2 kg or 0.9072 mt
1 lb = 16 oz = 0.4536 kg = 453.6 g

English Unit	Multiplied by	= Metric Unit
Ounce (oz)	28	grams (g)
Pound (lb)	0.4536	kilograms (kg)
Tons (t)	0.9072	metric tons (mt)

29 Understanding Journal Impact Factor and Citation Index

Vijay Prakash Mathur, Ashutosh Sharma

INTRODUCTION

During the past 3 to 4 decades, journals are being used for the evaluation of the research performance of academicians and researchers in all streams of science. The presumed quality of a defined set of journals is becoming the principle evaluation criteria due to various indices like Journal Impact Factor and citation index. Recent increase in the cost of scientific journals have also enthused the librarians to select a few 'good' journals using some yardstick. As a result, the academicians, researchers and librarian have to base their decisions on quantitative measures of assessing journal quality. The measures of assessing journal quality are also known as bibliometric indicators and have over the last 50 years become the chief quantitative measures of the quality of a journal, its research papers, the researchers who write these papers, and even the institute they work in. The aim of this chapter is to discuss the history of these quantitative measures of journalogy, its limitations and how these measures be used appropriately.

HISTORICAL BACKGROUND

The first attempt to rank scientific journals dates back to 1927 when Gross and Gross (1927) first reported use of counting references. However, the better scientific method for finding out the impact of the journal on scientific fraternity was first described by Garfield from the Institute of Scientific Information (ISI) in year 1955. But the term impact factor was not used until the publication of the 1961 Science Citation Index (SCI) in 1963. The inventors of SCI mentioned that highly cited large journals would be covered in the SCI, but some elite journals publishing mostly review articles would go unrecognized. Finally, the Journal Impact Factor (JIF) was created to help select journals for the

SCI and compare the journals regardless of their size. A biproduct of the SCI was the Journal Citation Reports (JCR) which was first published in the year 1975. The current JCR's have two editions covering journals in the areas of science, technology, and social sciences. The present day JCRs cover a more then 8000 journals from across the globe from 227 disciplines and 66 countries. The science stream including health sciences covers more than 6500 journals alone. Presently it has cited and citing journal statistics from year 1997 onwards.

METHOD OF CREATING JOURNAL CITATION REPORT

The electronic copies of all published journals are first obtained from publishers or hard copy is scanned using optical character recognition software. In order to properly index this database, few indicator fields like author, address, journal title, volume, year and page number, etc. are marked. Then a unique identifying code or tag is created by the computer for each paper. A similar unique code is also prepared for each of the references submitted at the end of each paper. These unique tags are then used for citation by matching. Thereby, with simple click of computer mouse, complete citation history of each article can be obtained.

SOME DEFINITIONS

Impact Factor

The impact factor is defined as: The number of times articles from a journal are cited within two years divided by the total number of articles published in the same journal during the two year period. The impact factor of a journal is intended to measure how often *on average* authors cite *moderately recent* articles from that particular journal.

$$2010 \text{ impact Factor} = \frac{\text{(All citations of 2008-2009 issues)}}{\text{(number of articles in the 2008-2009 issues)}}$$

The impact factor is a measure of the way a journal receives citations to its articles over time. The cumulative citations for two years tend to follow a curve and it rises sharply to a peak between two to six years after publication and then it declines exponentially. The citation curve of any journal can be described by the relative size of the curve in terms of area under the line, the extent to which the peak of the curve is close to the origin, and the rate of decline of the curve. The window period counted is 2 years.

Immediacy Index

The immediacy index of journal is intended to measure how often on average authors cite very recent articles from that particular journal and hence how rapidly the average paper from that journal is adopted into the literature. Immediacy index give a measure of skewness of the curve that is the extent to which the peak of the curve lies near to the origin of the graph.

Cited Half-life

The cited half-life is the calculated point (age in year) where 50% of the citations are under the age and 50% of the citations are over that age. The cited half life is a measure of the rate of decline of the citation curve. It is the number of years that the number of current citations takes to decline to 50% of its initial value. It is a measure of how long articles in a journal continue to be cited after publication.

Journal Impact Factor Versus other Bibliometric Indicators

The Impact factor has been under fire since several years and multiple authors have challenged the validity of the same. However, Xiu-fang WU et al (2008) and Tam Cam Ha et al (2006) and Kumar V et al (2009) have suggested that the comparison should be within the subject if we are using Impact factor for the quality of a publication. The Impact factor is a ratio where the numerator can be easily manipulated by changing some policies by the editor. Often the editors request the authors to use citation/references from their own journal and use limited number of references from outside the journal. Further few journals publishing more review articles tend to be cited more than other topic specific journals. Much controversy has been generated likewise on the use of this citation metric for ranking the quality of research of individuals and research groups. Despite of this, many biomedical scientists continue to pay attention to the impact factor based rankings and base their decisions on these.

Number of Authors and Impact Factor

The effect of the number of authors in a paper is closely connected to JIF, which varies from subject to subject. The number of authors are generally more in clinical sciences compared to the social sciences, since they require bigger team to plan, conduct, and analyze the data. Many of us have a tendency to cite own work by doing 'auto citation.' This practice usually distorts the true picture. Therefore, one should use ones sense of scientific propriety while citing ones own or parallel work.

Publication Type and Impact Factor

Within the same subject area there may also be a marked variation in the impact factor. This is being influenced by the type of the journal and the articles. In a sense 'impact factor' may be quite unintentionally 'tweaked' in rapid publication journals and articles of the current review type, why, because of a virtual deluge of papers published, it is but natural that the discerning reader is always on the lookout for a review on the topic of interest. Without doubt there is always a lot more information in a review than in original papers. Consequently, journals with a high number of reviews have an advantage in the impact factor league over those that published primary research papers. Furthermore, journals that are very selective or even restrictive can reduce the number of papers per issue and limit them to currently 'trendy' topics. This may be affecting their impact factor rating in a positive way.

Journal Size and Impact Factor

The size of the journal here means the number of articles published per annum, and the size of the measurement window which in case of the JCR is two years. For example, if a large number of journals (4000, arranged in quartiles based on size of journal) are examined and the mean variation in impact factor from one year to the next is plotted against size of the journal, there is a clear correlation between the extents of the impact factor fluctuation. This means, when impact factors are compared, journal size should always be taken into consideration.

Time Lag in Publication and Impact Factor

The time taken by the reviewers of a journal to assess a submitted research publication also affects the JIF because by definition, only previous 2 years publications are counted in JIF. In case one journal has longer gap between submission and publication due to waitlist/ longer review process, the reference may not be current by the time it is published. Since the impact factor calculation by the JCR works on a 2 years time frame, it really favors research that takes less time to complete. So the editors and the editorial board can make efforts to reduce the review time and enhance the publication time by using more and more electronic media and internet. However, the review process should be very rigorous and by no means there should be appalling quality.

Title/Abstract and the Impact Factor

The key words used for an article or the way of writing the abstract may also affect the cataloguing in the Journal Citation Reports (JCR). Sieck (2000) has tried to explain this phenomena by giving example of some words and phrases in title which are not true reprehensive of entire article. Therefore selection of key words is very important while writing the article.

Citation Half Life or Impact Factor

Also controversial is the fact that depending on the type of the publication, is it the impact factor rating or the cited half life of a publication that is more relevant? While impact factor only tells us about how many times an article has been cited, it is the 'cited half life' that according to some is more relevant. Citation half life is the number of publication years from the current year that accounts for 50 percent of current citations received. This citation metric provides an estimate of how long a publication will continue to impact the literature. Now one may ask, if the assessment of intellectual salience is being trivialized by the use of a system that has so many imperfections, then why are the journals that have the highest impact factors is considered 'the best'? Why is it always that a journal in which it is most difficult to have an article accepted has a high impact factor, if science should be judged by its content and not its wrapping then why undermine supplant true peer review? With so many questions the most suitable answers we believe were given by Hoeffel and Garfield who expressed the situation succinctly as follows: *"Impact factors are not a perfect tool to measure the quality of articles but there is nothing better and it has the advantage of already being in existence and is therefore, a good technique for scientific evaluation. Experience has shown that in each specialty the best journals are those in which it is most difficult to have an article accepted, and these are the journals that have a high impact factor. These journals existed long before the impact factor was devised. The use of impact factor as a measure of quality is widespread because it fits well with the opinion we have in each field of the best journals in our specialty. Finally Garfield "cautioned the use of impact factor to weigh the influence of a paper amounts to a prediction, albeit colored by probabilities".*

END NOTE

"Some part of this chapter has been copied verbatim from the article published in Indian Journal of Dental Research (Mathur VP, Sharma A.

Impact factor and other standardized measures of journal citation: A perspective. Indian J Dent Res 2009;20(1):81-5) with permission."

SUGGESTED READING

1. Adam D. The counting house. Nature 2002;415:726-9.
2. Adams KM. Impact factors: Aiming at the wrong target. Cortex 2001;37(4): 600-3.
3. Buchtel HA. Libraries and the Academy (editorial). Cortex 2001; 37(4): 455-6.
4. Davis PM. "Where to spend our e-journal money? Defining a university library's core collection through citation analysis." John Hopkins University Press, Baltimore, USA 2002;2(1):155-66.
5. Gannon F. The impact of the impact factor (editorial). EMBO Reports 2000; 1(4):293.
6. Garfield E. How cam impact factors be improved? Br Med J 1996;313:411-3.
7. Garfield E. Journal impact factor: a brief review. CMAJ 1999;161(8):979-80.
8. Hoeffel C. Journal impact factors (letter). Allergy 1998;53:1225.
9. Kumar V, Upadhyay S, Medhi B. Impact of the "impact factor" in biomedical research: its use and misuse. Singapore Med J 2009;50:752-5.
10. Linde A. On the pitfalls of journal ranking by impact factor (editorial). Eur J Oral Sci 1998;106:525-6.
11. Martin-Sempere MJ, Rey-rocha J and Garzon-Garcia B. Assessing quality of domestic scientific journals in genographically oriented disciplines: scientists' judgments versus citations. Research Evaluation 2002; 11(4):149-54.
12. Opthof T. Submission, acceptance rate, rapid review system and impact factor (editorial). Cardiovascular Research 1999;41:1-4.
13. Seglen PO. Citations and journal impact factors: questionable indicators of research quality (review). Allergy 1997;52:1050-6.
14. Tam Cam Ha, Say Beng Tan, Khee Chee Soo. The Journal Impact factor: too much of an impact. Ann Acad Med Singapore 2006;35:911-6.
15. Xiu-fng WU, Qiang FU, Ronald ROUSSEAU. On indexing in the web of science and predicting Journal impact factor. J Zhejiang Univ Sci B 2008;9:582-90.

30 Frequently Asked Questions

Kandaswamy Deivanayagam

It is a good trend that the awareness has increased amongst the academicians, regarding the importance of publications in reputed index journals. The fact that publications are necessary for promotions, also makes it mandatory for the aspiring teachers to go to the next level. But the basis for any good publication is a well documented case report of interest or a proper study with the right protocol. The following are a few frequently asked questions regarding publication.

1. I have absolutely no idea how to publish an article so where do I begin?

Answer: Most of us complete a study and then think of publishing it but the right thing to do would be to choose that a topic of study which would be applicable from publication point of view. Choose a topic which has relevance and has not been reported and has some significance in the literature. Remember that repeated studies or already concluded studies will not be accepted for publication.

2. How will I select a topic for a study which would be worthy of publication?

Answer: In my opinion, I have always looked for the existing lacunae in our knowledge.

I would give an example from dental point of view. Whenever I used to teach about vitality test of a tooth, I used to say the ideal way to test the vitality of a tooth is to study the blood flow, however in present scenario we are only testing the nerve stimulation. Pulp oximetry can be used for measuring the blood flow. When I studied further, I realized that pulse oximetry is not effective on the teeth because of a simple drawback that the existing sensor could not be placed parallel to each other (which is mandatory) over the tooth. Then, we designed a holder which can hold the existing ear lobe sensor of pulse oximetry parallel to each other when placed over the tooth. We have 3 indexed publications on this design. So it is always better to look for lacunae in the existing knowledge.

3. How to select the most accepted methodology for a study?

Answer: It is mandatory that you keep in touch with the recent articles that are published in reputed indexed journals which will give us the accepted methodology for the selected topic.

For example: Many studies get rejected on the basis of methodology. The editor usually requests to refer their previous editorials in which the editorial team of the journal has decided not to accept that methodology anymore. It is not only important to read the articles in the journals but also the editorials. You can also use a methodology not tried before but you have to make sure that it is an appropriate for that particular problem.

4. How many variables can we select for a study and how to know the correct sample size?

Answer: The more the number of variables, the more difficult it is to compare and discuss. It is always easier to select one particular aspect as a variable keeping the remaining parameters standardized. The most important point to keep in mind is after we decide on the number of variables; the study should be discussed with the statistician. He/she alone can decide on the sample size and also the type of statistical analysis to be employed.

5. What are positive control and negative control?

Answer: It is always preferable to have a positive and a negative control for the study.

For example: In a study comparing the antibacterial efficiency of irrigants, the following materials were used as irrigants namely propolis, betadine, morinda citrifolia, chlorhexidine and saline. Here the positive control is chlorhexidine and the negative control is saline.

6. Should the results be tabulated or should it be interpreted also?

Answer: It is also necessary to interpret the results by saying which material has performed better in ascending or descending order with the groups having a statistically significant difference.

7. How to select the journal for the publication of my study?

Answer: The selection of the journal depends on the nature of the study. You need to select a journal in such a way that the study will fall into their main purview.

For example: If you want to submit a case report, you must be able to select a journal which will accept case reports. So you select a journal which gives you the best chance of publishing your article.

8. How do I know the right format to write my article?

Answer: The format varies from one journal to another and once you have selected the journal, read the instructions to the author first, that will give you a fair idea as to how to write your article.

9. What should I write in the introduction?

Hint—Please refer chapter 9 for details

Answer: Introduce the readers to the existing concepts or techniques and highlight the short comings or the lacunae on how your study will address this area. An ideal introduction should be of 2 to 3 paragraph and divided into two components namely background. The first paragraph describes the natured problem or issue. The second paragraph should elaborate on the importance of the problem. The third paragraph should describe the rationale (reason/purpose) of the current study and contain the research question and the hypothesis and state, how it relates to previous work.

10. In writing the methodology, what are those important factors which I must be kept in mind?

Hint — Please refer chapter 10 for details

Answer: The important things one should keep in mind is that if you are using any materials, the year and date of manufacturing, batch number, the place of manufacturer, and the company of the manufacturer should be mentioned in the form of a table.

If the study involves any ethical clearance, then it should be included in the methodology. Every procedure should be explained in detail in the methodology, if any equipment is used the approved protocol for using the equipment along with the principle behind the equipment should be mentioned. As much as possible, it is better to use the internationally accepted protocols and the type of protocol followed should be mentioned instead of simply writing the material that has been used as per the manufacturer's direction.

It is better to explain the step by step procedure and then mention that it is according to manufacturer's instruction. If possible a small summary of the procedure preferably in the form of a flowchart can be given at the end.

11. What points I must keep in mind in writing the discussion?

Hint— Please refer chapter 15 for details

Answer: Usually the first part of discussion should revolve around the need for your study and the reasons for using a particular methodology or materials. The second part of the study should discuss the results for the study.

12. How many references should my study have?

Answer: It is not the number of references that matter but the references which are quoted must be apt for the concept of your discussion. Never write that there are numerous studies and various authors to indicate a particular concept instead quote references of specific articles which substantiate your claim.

You must keep in mind that the reviewer of your article has access to all your references and they will go through each and every reference you have quoted to check its authenticity and the content. Avoid giving references in which you have access only to the abstract and not to the full article.

13. If my article is rejected by a journal what do I do next?

Hint — Please refer chapter 24 for details

Answer: Quite a few people tell me that their article is rejected by an international journal and whether they could send it to a National journal. When an article is rejected, first read the editor's comments. If the editor's comment says the article is not within its scope, then we can look for the journal which probably will have an interest in your topic. If the editor's note says that the article is rejected based on the reviewer's comments, then go through the reviewer's comments carefully. If you can successfully answer and defend all the queries raised by the reviewers, then you can think of sending it to another journal.

A good English is mandatory for any international publication so it is preferable to give your article to an English teacher to check the language before sending it for publication. I personally maintain a file for the reviewer's comments of my rejected articles. And everytime I send a new article for publication I refer to this file to check if I have overlooked any particular point.

Before starting any new study there are a few things you should keep in mind. I will not approve a study which is going to end with a conclusion that the results of the study is in concurrence with studies done by x,y,z (It simply means you are only adding number to the existence studies on the same topic.) or further studies are required to prove the same point (that means you are not definitive and conclusive). Any study should be able to conclude decisively on the selected research question.

14. What is plagiarism?

Answer: "Plagiare"—to steal
• It is intellectual theft and is a serious scientific misconduct

15. What are the common types of plagiarism?

Answer: Following are the common types of plagiarism
• Word for word—without putting inquotes

- Paraphrasing without citing reference
- Plagiarism of ideas
- Plagiarism of authorship

16. Why do people plagiarize?

Answer: People plagiarize due to Ignorance, Lack of knowledge on the ethics of scholarly writing, Ambition, Fierce competition, Pressure from seniors, Publish or perish system, Poor writing skills and to be faster.

17. How to avoid plagiarism?

Answer   • If you use something word for word it must be acknowledged
- For short quotes, use quotation marks in the sentence
- For longer quotes indent the entire passage
- If you have used a table, chart, diagram, etc. cite the source directly below
- It is not enough to have cited the reference somewhere in the text.

Before I conclude, I would like to say there is no greater joy than seeing your study in print in a reputed journal.
Let me wish you all a joyful publication.

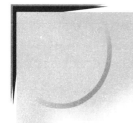

Appendices

Selected Journal Title Word Abbreviations*

Word	Abbreviation	Word	Abbreviation
Abstracts	Abstr.	Bacteriology	Bacteriol.
Academy	Acad.	Bakteriologie	Bakteriol.
Acta	No abbrev.	Berichte	Ber.
Advances	Adv.	Biochemical	Biochem.
Agricultural	Agric.	Biochemica	Biochim.
American	Am.	Biological	Biol.
Anales	An.	Biologie	Biol.
Analytical	Anal	Botanical	Bot.
Anatomical	Anat.	Botanisches	Bot.
Annalen	Ann.	Botany	Bot.
Annales	Ann.	British	Br.
Annals	Ann.	Bulletin	Bull.
Annual	Annu.	Bureau	Bur.
Anthropological	Anthropol.	Canadian	Can.
Antibiotic	Antibiot.	Cardiology	Cardiol.
Antimicrobial	Antimicrob.	Cell	No abbrev.
Applied	Appl.	Cellular	Cell.

Contd....

* Reproduced with permission from— Robert A Day. Appendix 1, Selected Journal Title
Word Abbreviations. In: Robert A Day(ed) How to write and publish a scientific paper. 4th
edn. ABC-CLIO Press Santa Barbara, California, USA; 1995. pp. 187-9.

Contd....

Arbeiten	Arb.	Central	Cent.
Archive	Arch.	Chemical	Chem.
Archives	Arch.	Chemie	Chem.
Archivio	Arch.	Chemistry	Chem.
Association	Assoc.	Chemotherapy	Chemother.
Astronomical	Astron.	Chimie	Chim.
Atomic	At.	Clinical	Clin.
Australian	Aust.	Commonwealth	Commw.
Bacteriological	Bacterial.	Comptes	c.
		Conference	Conf.
Contributions	Contrib.	Immunity	Immune.
Current	Curr.	Immunology	Immunol.
Dairy	No abbrev.	Industrial	Ind.
Dental	Dent.	Institute	Inst.
Developmental	Dev.	Internal	Intern.
Diseases	Dis.	International	Int.
Drug	No abbrev.	Jahrbuch	Jahrb.
Ecology	Ecol.	Jahresberichte	Jahresber.
Economics	Econ.	Japan, Japanese	Jpn.
Edition	Ed.	Journal	J.
Electric	Electr.	Laboratory	Lab.
Electrical	Electr.	Magazine	Mag.
Engineering	Eng.	Material	Matr.
Entomologia	Entomol.	Mathematics	Math.
Entomologica	Entomol.	Mechanical	Mech.
Entomological	Entomol.	Medical	Med.
Environmental	Environ.	Medicine	Med.
Ergebnisse	Ergeb.	Methods	No abbrev.
Ethnology	Ethnol.	Microbiological	Microbiol.
European	Eur.	Microbiology	Microbiol.
Exceropta	No abbrev.	Monographs	Monogr.
Experimental	Exp.	Monthly	Mon.

Contd....

Contd....

Fauna	No abbrev.	Morphology	Morphol.
Federal	Fed.	National	Natl.
Federation	Fed.	Natural, nature	Nat.
Fish	No abbrev.	Neurology	Neurol.
Fisheries	Fish.	Nuclear	Nucl.
Flora	No abbrev.	Nutrition	Nutr.
Folia	No abbrev.	Obstetrical	Obstet.
Food	No abbrev.	Official	Off.
Forest	For.	Organic	Org.
Forschung	Forsch.	Paleontology	Paleontol.
Fortschritte	Fortschr.	Pathology	Pathol.
Freshwater	No abbrev.	Pharmacology	Pharmacol.
Gazette	Gaz.	Philosophical	Philos.
General	Gen.	Physical	Phys.
Genetics	Genet.	Physik	Phys.
Geographical	Geogr.	Physiology	Physiol.
Geological	Geol.	Pollution	Pollut.
Geologische	Geol.	Proceedings	Proc.
Gesellschaft	Ges.	Psychological	Psycho.
Helvetica	Helv.	Publications	Publ.
History	Hist.	Quarterly	Q
Rendus	R.	Technik	Tech.
Report	Rep.	Technology	Technol.
Research	Res.	Therapeutics	Ther.
Review	Rev.	Transactions	Trans.
Revue, Revista	Rev.	Tropical	Trop.
Rivista	Riv.	United States	U.S.
Royal	R.	University	Univ.
Scandinavian	Scand.	Untersuchung	Unters.
Science	Sci.	Urological	Urol.
Scientific	Sci.	Verhandlungen	Verh.
Series	Ser.	Veterinary	Vet.

Contd....

Contd....

Service	Serv.	Virology	Virol.
Society	Soc.	Vitamin	Vitam.
Special	Spec.	Wissenschaftliche	Wiss.
Station	Stn.	Zeitschrift	Z.
Studies	Stud.	Zentralblatt	Zentralbl.
Surgery	Surg.	Zoologie	Zool.
Survey	Surv.	Zoology	Zool.
Symposia	Symp.		
Symposium	Symp.		
Systematic	Syst.		
Technical	Tech.		

APPENDIX 2

Abbreviations that may be Used Without Definition in Table*

Term	Abbreviation	Term	Abbreviation
Amount	Amt	Specific activity	sp act
Approximately	Approx	Specific gravity	sp gr
Average	Avg	Standard deviation	SD
Concentration	Concn	Standard error	SE
Diameter	Diam	Standard error of the mean	SEM
Experiment	Expt	Temperature	temp
Experimental	Exptl	Versus	vs
Height	Ht	Volume	vol
Molecular weight	mol wt	Week	wk
Number	no.	Weight	wt
Preparation	Prepn	Year	yr

* Reproduced with permission from—Robert A Day. Appendix 2, Abbreviations That May Be Used Without Definition in Table Headings. In:Robert A Day(ed) How to write and publish a scientific paper. 4th edn. ABC-CLIO Press Santa Barbara, California, USA; 1995. p. 190.

APPENDIX 3

Common Errors in Style and in Spelling*

Wrong	Right
Acetyl-glucosamine	Acetylglucosamine
Acid fast bacteria	Acid-fast bacteria
Acid fushsin	Acid fuchsine
Acridin orange	Acridine orange
Acriflavin	Acriflavine
Aesculin	Esculin
Airborn	Airborne
Air-flow	Airflow
Ampoule	Ampoule
Analogous	Analogous
Analize	Analyze
Bacteristatic	Bacteriostatic
Baker's yeast	Bakers' yeast
Bi-monthly	Bimonthly
Bio–assay	Bioassay
Biurette	Biuret
Blendor	Blender
Blood sugar	Blood glucose
Bromcresol blue	Bromocresol blue
By-pass	Bypass
Byproduct	By-product
Can not	Cannot
Catabolic repression	Catabolite repression
Chloracetic	Chloroacetic
Clearcut	Clear-cut
Colicine	Colicin
Coverslip	Cover slip
Co-worker	Coworker

Contd....

* *Reproduced with permission from— Robert A Day. Appendix 3, Common Errors in Style and in Spelling. In:Robert A Day(ed) How to write and publish a scientific paper; 4th edn. ABC-CLIO Press Santa Barbara, California, USA; 1995. pp. 191-4.*

Contd....

Cross over (n.)	Crossover
Crossover (v.)	Cross over
Darkfield	Dark field
Data is	Data are
Desoxy-	Deoxy-
Dessicator	Desiccators
Dialise	Dialyze
Disc	Disk
Ehrlenmeyer flask	Erlenmeyer flask
Electronmicrograph	Electron micrograph
Electrophorese	Subject to electrophoresis
Fermenter (apparatus)	Fermentor
Fermentor (organism)	Fermenter
Ferridoxin	Ferredoxin
Fluorite	Fluorite
Fluorescent antibody technique	Fluorescent-antibody technique
Fungous (n)	Fungus
Fungus (adj.)	Fungous
Gelatin	Gelatin
Germ-free	Germfree
Glucose-6-phosphate	Glucose 6-phosphate
Glycerin	Glycerol
Glycollate	Glycolate
Gonnorhea	Gonorrhea
Gram-negative	Gram-negative
Gram stain	Gram stain
Gyrotory	Gyratory
Halflife	Half-life
Haptene	Hapten
Hela cells	HeLa cells
Hep-2-cells	HEp-2 cells
Herpes virus	Herpesvirus

Contd....

Contd....

Hydrolize	Hydrolyze
Hydrolyzate	Hydrolysate
Immunofluorescent techniques	Immunofluorescence techniques
India ink	India ink
Indol	Idole
Innocula	Inocula
Iodimetric	Iodometric
Ion exchange resin	Ion-exchange resin
Isocitritase	Isocitratase
Keiselguhr	Kieselguhr
Large concentration	High concentration
Less data	Fewer data
Leucocyte	Leukocyte
Little data	Few data
Low quantity	Small quantity
Mediums	Media
Melanin	Melanin
Merthiolate	Merthiolate
Microphotograph	Photomicrograph
Mid-point	Midpoint
Moiety	Moiety
Much data	Many data
New-born	Newborn
Occurrence	Occurrence
Over-all	Overall
Papergram	Paper chromatogram
Paraffine	Paraffin
Petri dish	Petri dish
Phenolsulfophthalein	Phenolsulfonephthalein
Phosphorous (n.)	Phosphorus
Phosphorus (adj.)	Phosphorous
Planchette	Planchet

Contd....

Contd....

Plexiglass	Plexiglas
Post-mortem	Postmortem
Pyocine	Pyocin
Pyrex	Pyrex
Radio-active	Radioactive
Regime	Regimen
Re-inoculate	Reinoculate
Saltwater	Salt water
Sea water	Seawater
Selfinoculate	Self-inoculate
Semi-complete	Semicomplete
Shelflife	Shelf life
Sidearm	Side arm
Small concentration	Low concentration
Spore-forming	Sporeforming
Stationary phase culture	Stationary-phase culture
Step-wise	Stepwise
Students' T test	Student's t test
Sub-inhibitory	Subinhibitory
T^2 phase	T2 phase
Technic	Technique
Teflon	Teflon
Thioglycollate	Thioglycolate
Thyroxin	Thyroxine
Transfered	Transferred
Transferring	Transferring
Transferable	Transferable
Trichloracetic acid	Trichloroacetic acid
Tris-(hydroxymethy) Amino-methane	Tris(hydroxymethyl) Aminomethane
Trypticase	Trypticase
Tryptophane	Tryptophan
Ultra-sound	Ultrasound

Contd....

Contd....

Un-tested	Untested
Urinary infection	Urinary tract infection
Varying amounts of cloudiness	Varying cloudiness
Varying concentrations (5, 10, 15 mg/ml)	Various concentrations (5, 10, 15mg/ml)
Waterbath	Water bath
Wave length	Wavelength
X ray (adj.)	X-ray
X-ray (n.)	X ray
Zero-hour	Zero hour

APPENDIX 4

Words and Expressions to Avoid*

Jargon	*Preferred Usage*
A considerable amount of	Much
A considerable number of	Many
A decreased amount of	Less
A decreased number of	Fewer
A majority of	Most
A number of	Many
A small number of	A few
Absolutely essential	Essential
Accounted for by the fact	Because
Adjacent to	Near
Along the lines of	Like
An adequate amount of	Enough
An example of this is the fact that	For example
An order of magnitude faster	10 times faster
Apprise	Inform
Are of the same opinion	Agree
As a consequence of	Because
As a matter of fact	In fact (or leave out)
As a result of	Because
As is the case	As happens
As of this date	Today

* *Reproduced with permission from— Robert A Day. Appendix 4, Words and Expressions to Avoid, In:Robert A Day(ed) How to write and publish a scientific paper. 4th edn. ABC-CLIO Press Santa Barbara, California, USA; 1995. pp. 195-200.*

As to	About (or leave out)
At a rapid rate	Rapidly
At an earlier date	Previously
At an early date	Soon
At no time	Never
At some future time	Later
At the conclusion of	After
At the present time	Now
At this point in time	Now
Based on the fact that	Because
Because of the fact that	Because
By means of	By, with
Causal factor	Cause
Cognizant of	Aware of
Completely full	Full
Consensus of opinion	Consensus
Considerable amount of	Much
Contingent upon	Dependent on
Definitely proved	Proved
Despite the fact that	Although
Due to the fact that	Because
During the course of	During, while
During the time that	While
Effectuate	Cause
Elucidate	Explain
Employ	Use
Enclosed herewith	Enclosed
End result	Result
Endeavor	Try
Entirely eliminate	Eliminate
Eventuate	Happen
Fabricate	Make
Facilitate	Help
Fatal outcome	Death
Fewer in number	Fewer
Finalize	End
First of all	First
Following	After
For the purpose of	For
For the reason that	Since, because
From the point of view of	For
Future plans	Plans
Give an account of	Describe

Give rise to	Cause
Has been engaged in a study of	Has studied
Has the capability of	Can
Have the appearance of	Look like
Having regard to	About
Immune serum	Antiserum
Impact (v.)	Affect
Implement	Start, put into action
In a number of cases	Some
In a position to	Can, may
In a satisfactory manner	Satisfactorily
In a situation in which	When
In a very real sense	In a sense (or leave out)
In almost all instances	Nearly always
In case	If
In close proximity to	Close, near
In connection with	About, concerning
In light of the fact that	Because
In many cases	Often
In only a small number of cases	Rarely
In order to	To
In relation to	Toward, to
In respect to	About
In some cases	Sometimes
In terms of	About
In the absence of	Without
In the event that	If
In the not-too-distant future	Soon
In the possession of	Has, have
In this day and age	Today
In view of the fact that	Because, since
Inasmuch as	For, as
Incline to the view	Think
Initiate	Begin, start
Is defined as	Is
Is desirous of	Wants
It has been reported by smith	Smith reported
It is crucial that	Must
It is doubtful that	Possibly
It is evident that a produced b	A produced b
It is generally believed	Many think
It is of interest to note that	Leave out
It is often the case that	Often
It is suggested that	I think

Of the opinion that	Think that
On a daily basis	Daily
On account of	Because
On behalf of	For
On no occasion	Never
On the basis of	By
On the grounds that	Since, because
On the part of	By, among, for
On those occasions in which	When
Should it prove the case that	If
Smaller in size	Smaller
So as to	To
Subject matter	Subject
Subsequent to	After
Sufficient	Enough
Take into consideration	Consider
Terminate	End
The great majority of	Most
The opinion is advanced that	I think
The predominate number of	Most
The question as to whether	Whether
The reason is because	Because
The vast majority of	Most
There is reason to believe	I think
They are the investigators who	They
What is the explanation of	Why
With a view to	To
With reference to	About (or leave out)
With regard to	Concerning, about (or leave out)
With respect to	About
With the possible exception of	Except
With the result that	So that
Within the realm of possibility	Possible

APPENDIX 5

Prefix and Abbreviations for SI (Systeme International) Units*

No.	Prefix	Abbreviation
10^{-18}	atto	a
10^{-15}	femto	f
10^{-12}	pico	p
10^{-9}	nano	n
10^{-6}	micro	μ
10^{-3}	milli	m
10^{-2}	centi	c
10^{-1}	deci	d
10	deka	da
10^{2}	hecto	h
10^{3}	kilo	k
10^{6}	mega	M
10^{9}	giga	G
10^{12}	tera	T
10^{15}	peta	P
10^{18}	exa	E

APPENDIX 6

Accepted Abbreviations and Symbols**

Term	Abbreviation or Symbol
Absorbance	A
Acetyl	Ac
Adenine	Ade
Adenosine	Ado
Adenosine 5′ – diphosphate	ADP
Adenosine 5′ – monophosphate	AMP
Adenosine 5- triphosphate	ATP

Contd...

---

* *Reproduced with permission from — Robert A Day. Appendix 5, Prefixes and Abbreviations for SI (Systeme International) Units. In:Robert A Day(ed) How to write and publish a scientific paper. 4th edn. ABC-CLIO Press Santa Barbara, California, USA; 1995. pp. 201.*

** *Reproduced with permission from — Robert A Day. Appendix 6, Accepted Abbreviations and Symbols. In:Robert A Day(ed) How to write and publish a scientific paper. 4th edn. ABC-CLIO Press Santa Barbara, California, USA; 1995. pp 202-4.*

Contd...

Adenosine triphosphatase	ATPase
Alanine	Ala
Alternating current	ac
Ampere	A
Antibody	Ab
Antigen	Ag
Arabinose	Ara
Bacilli Calmette-Guerin	BCG
Becquerel	Bq
Biological oxygen demand	BOD
Blood urea nitrogen	BUN
Boiling point	bp
Candela	cd
Central nervous system	CNS

Coenzyme a	CoA
Coulomb	C
Counts per minute	cpm
Cytidine	Cyd
Cytidine 5′ – diphosphate	CDP
Cytidine 5′ – monophosphate	CMP
Cytidine 5′ – triphosphate	CTP
Cytosine	Cyt
Degree celsius	°C
Deoxyribonuclease	DNase
Deoxyribonucleic acid	DNA
Deoxyuridine monophosphate	DUMP
Diethylaminoethyl cellulose	DEAE-cellulose
Electrocardiogram	ECG
Electroencephalogram	EEG
Ethyl	Et
Ethylene diamine tetra acetate	EDTA
Farad	F
Flavin adenine dinucleotide	FAD

Flavin mononucleotide	FMN
Gauss	G
Gram	g
Gravity	g .
Guanidine	Gdn
Guanine	Gua
Guanosine	Guo
Guanosine 5′ – diphosphate	GDP
Hemoglobin	Hb
Hemoglobin, oxygenated	HbO_2
Henry	H
Heptyl	Hp
Hertz	Hz
Hexyl	Hx
Horsepower	hp
Hour	h
Infrared	IR
Inosine 5′ – diphosphate	IDP
International unit	IU
Intravenous	i.v.
Isoleucyl	Ile
Joule	J
Kelvin	K
Kilogram	Kg
Kinetic energy	KE
Lethal dose, median	LD_{50}
Leucyl	Leu
Litre (liter)	l
Lumen	lm
Lux	lx
Lysinyl	Lys
Melting point	mp
Messenger ribo-nucleic acid	mRNA
Meta-methionyl	m-Met
Methyl	Me
Metre (meter)	m

Michaelis constant	K_m
Milliequivalent	meq
Minimum lethal dose	MLD
Minute (time)	min
Molar (concentration)	M
Mole	mol
Muramic acid	Mur
Newton	N
Nicotinamide adenine dinucleotide	NAD
Second (time)	s
Serum glutamic oxalacetic transaminase	SGOT
Seryl	Ser
Siemens	S
Species	sp.(sing.), spp. (pl.)
Specific gravity	sp gr
Standard deviation	SD
Standard error	SE
Standard temperature and pressure	STP
Steradian	sr
Subcutaneous	s.c.
Tesla	T
Tobacco mosaic virus	TMV
Tone (metric ton)	t
Transfer ribonucleic acid	tRNA
Tris (hydroxyl methyl) aminomethane	Tris
Tyrosinyl	Tyr
Ultraviolet	UV
United states pharmacopeia	USP
Uracil	Ura
Uridine 5' – diphosphate	UDP
Volt	V
Volume	V
Watt	W
Weber	Wb
Week	wk
White blood cells (leukocytes)	WBC
Xanthine	Xan
Xanthosine	Xao
Xanthosine 5' – diphosphate	XDP
Xylose	xyl
Year	yr

TERMINOLOGIES*

Abstract—Brief synopsis of a paper, usually providing a summary of each major section of the paper. Different from a summary, which is usually a summary of conclusions.

Acknowledgments—The section of a paper (following the Discussion but preceding References) designed to give thanks to individuals and organizations for the help, advice, or financial assistance they provided during the research and during the writing of the paper.

Ad hoc reviewer—See Referee.

Address—Identifies the author and supplies the author's mailing address.

Alphabet-number system—A system of literature citation in which references are arranged alphabetically in References or Literature Cited, numbered, and then cited by number in the text. A variation of the name and year system.

Archival journal—This term is equivalent to "primary journal" and refers to a journal that publishes original research results.

Author—A person who actively contributed to the design and execution of the experiments and who takes intellectual responsibility for the research results being reported.

Biological Abstracts—The largest and best-known repository (in the form of abstracts) of knowledge in biology. Published by Biosciences Information Service.

Camera-ready copy— Anything that is suitable for photographic reproduction in a book or journal without the need for typesetting. Authors often supply complicated formulas, chemical structures, flowcharts, etc. as camera-ready copy to avoid the necessity of proofreading and the danger of error in typesetting.

Caption—See Legend.

CBE—See Council of Biology Editors.

Chemical Abstracts—The largest and best-known repository (in the form of abstracts) of knowledge in chemistry. Published by the American Chemical Society.

Citation-order system—A system of referencing in which references are cited in numerical order as they appear in the text. Thus, references is in citation order, not in alphabetical order.

Coeditor—The title given to a person (usually an employee of the publisher) whose responsibility it is to prepare manuscripts for publication by providing markup for the printer as well as any needed improvements in spelling, grammar, and style.

Compositor—One who sets type. Equivalent terms are "typesetter" and "keyboarder".

Conference report—A paper written for presentation at a conference. Most conference reports do not meet the definition of valid publication. A well-written

---

* *Reproduced with permission from— Robert A Day. Glossary of Technical terms. In:Robert A Day(ed) How to write and publish a scientific paper. 4th edn. ABC-CLIO Press Santa Barbara, California, USA; 1995. pp. 205-210.*

conference report can and should be short; experimental detail and literature citation should be kept to a minimum.

Copyeditor or Technical editor—The person who is responsible for changing the accepted papers into the journal's style, he edits the language and checks for completeness, consistency, paginate the manuscript etc.

Copyright—The exclusive legal rights to reproduce, publish, and sell written intellectual property OR It is a law that protects writers from having their work copied without permission.

Corresponding author—The author whose full contact details appear on a publication and who is the point of contact with the journal for handling reviewer's comments.

Council of Biology Editors—An organization whose members are involved with the writing, editing, and publishing of book and journals in biology and related fields.

Cropping—The marking of a photograph so as to indicate parts that need not appear in the published photograph. As a result, the essential material is "enlarged" and highlighted.

Current Contents—A weekly publication providing photographic reproductions of the contents pages of many journals. Scientists can thus keep up with what is being published in their field. Six different editions are published in different fields (including Arts and Humanities) by the Institute for Scientific Information.

Discussion—The final section of an IMRAD paper. Its purpose is to fit the results from the current study into the preexisting fabric of knowledge. The important points will be expressed as conclusions.

Dual publication—Publication of the same data two (or more) times in primary journals. A clear violation of scientific ethics.

Editor —The title usually given to the person who decides what will (and will not) be published in a journal or in a multiauthor book.

Editorial consultant—See Referee

Festschrift—A volume of writings by different authors presented as a tribute or memorial to a particular individual.

Galley proof—See Proof

Graph—Lines, bars, or other pictorial representations of data. Graphs are useful for showing the trends and directions of data. If exact values must be listed, a table is usually superior.

Hackneyed expression—An overused, stale, or trite expression.

Halftone—A photoengraving made from an image photographed through a screen and then etched so that the details of the image are reproduced in dots.

Hard copy—When an old-fashioned manuscript on paper is provided via a word processor or computer, it is called "hard copy".

Harvard system—See Name and year system.

Impact factor—A basis for judging the quality of journals. A journal with a high impact factor (the average number of citations per article published, as determined by the Science Citation Index) is apparently used more than a journal with a low impact factor.

IMRAD—An acronym derived from Introduction, Methods, Results, and Discussion, the organizational scheme of most modern scientific papers.

Incunabula—Books printed between 1455 and 1500 A.D.

Introduction—The first section of an IMRAD paper. Its purpose is to state clearly the problem investigated and to provide the reader with relevant background information.

Jargon—Webster's Tenth New Collegiate Dictionary defines jargon as "a confused unintelligible language".

Keyboarder—See Compositor.

Legend—The title or name given to an illustration, along with explanatory information about the illustration. Usually, this material should not be lettered on a graph or photograph. It will be typeset neatly by the compositor and positioned below the illustration. Also called a "caption".

Literature Cited—The heading used by many journals to list references cited in an article. The headings "References" and (rarely) "Bibliography" are also used.

Managing Editor—A title often given to the person who manages the business affairs of a journal. Typically, the managing editor is not involved with editing (acceptance of manuscripts) but is responsible for copyediting (part of the production process).

Markup for the Typesetter—Marks and symbols used by copyeditors (and sometimes authors, as in underlining for italics) to transmit type specifications to the typesetter.

Masthead statement—A statement by the publisher, usually given on the title page of the journal, giving ownership of the journal and a succinet statement describing the purpose and scope of the journal.

Materials and Methods—See Methods.

Methods—The second section of an IMRAD paper. Its purpose is to describe the experiment in such detail that a competent colleague could repeat the experiment and obtain the same or equivalent results.

Monograph—A specialized, detailed book written by specialists for other specialists.

Name and year system—A system of referencing in which a reference is cited in the text by the last name of the author and the year of publication, e.g. Smith (1990). Also known as the Harvard system.

Offprints—See Reprints.

Oral report—Similar in organization to a published paper, except that it lacks experimental detail and extensive literature citation.

Peer review—Review of a manuscript by peers of the author (scientists working in the same area of specialization) OR It is a formal system whereby a piece of academic work is scrutinized by people who were not involved in its creation but are considered knowledgeable in the subject.

Plagiarism—Plagiarism is defined as "using someone else's words, ideas or results without attribution.

Primary journal—A journal that publishes original research results.

Primary publication—The first publication of original research results, in a form whereby peers of the author can repeat the experiments and test the conclusions, and in a journal or other source document readily available within the scientific community.

Printer—Historically, a device that prints or a person who prints. Often, however, "printer" is used to mean the printing company and is used as shorthand for all of the many occupations involved in the printing process, e.g. compositors, press operators, plate-makers, and binders. A distinctly different meaning of "printer" is "computer printer", a device attached to a computer for the purpose of "printing hard copy" (supplying the computer output on paper).

Proof—A copy of typeset material sent to authors, editors, or managing editors for correction of typographical errors. Unpaged proofs are called "galley proofs"; paged proofs are called "page proofs".

Proofreaders' marks—A set of marks and symbols used to instruct the compositor regarding errors on proofs.

Publisher—A person or organization handling the business activities concerned with publishing a book of journal.

Referee—A person, usually a peer of the author, asked to examine a manuscript and advise the editor regarding publication. The term "reviewer" is used more frequently but perhaps with less exactness.

Reprints—Separately printed journal articles supplied to authors (usually for a fee). These reprints (sometimes called offprints) are widely circulated among scientists.

Results—The third section of an IMRAD paper. Its purpose is to present the new information gained in the study being reported.

Review paper—A paper written to review a number of previously published primary papers. Such reviews can be simply annotated references in a particular field, or they can be critical, interpretive studies of the literature in a particular field.

Reviewer—See Referee.

Running head—A headline repeated on consecutive pages of a book or journal. The titles of articles in journals are often shortened and used as running heads. Also called running headlines.

Science writing—A type of writing whose purpose is to communicate scientific knowledge to a wide audience including (usually) both scientists and nonscientists.

Scientific paper—A written and published report describing original research results.

Scientific writing—A type of writing whose purpose is to communicate new scientific findings to other scientists.

Series titles—Titles of articles published as a series over the course of time. These titles have a main title common to all papers in the series and a subtitle (usually introduced with a roman numeral) specific for each paper.

Society for Scholarly Publishing—An organization of scholars, editors, publishers, librarians, printers, booksellers, and others engaged in scholarly publishing.

Summary—Usually a summary of conclusions, placed at the end of a paper. Different from an Abstract, which usually summarizes all major parts of a paper and which appears at the beginning of the paper (heading abstract).

Syntax—The order of words within phrases, clauses, and sentences.

Table—Presentation of (usually) numbers in columnar form. Tables are used when many determinations need be presented and the exact numbers have importance. If only "the shape of the data" is important, a graph is usually preferable.

Thesis—A manuscript demanded of an advanced-degree candidate; its purpose is to prove that the candidate is capable of doing original research. The term "dissertation" is essentially equivalent but should be reserved for a manuscript submitted for a doctorate.

Title—The fewest possible words that adequately describe the contents of a paper, book, poster, etc.

Trade books—Books sold primarily through the book trade (book whole-salers and retailers) to the general public. Most scientific books, on the other hand, are sold primarily by direct mail.

Type composition—The typing (keyboarding) of the manuscript of the publisher in accord with the markup for the compositor provided by the copy editor.

Typesetter—See Compositor.

Index